T0201999

OXFORD STUDIES IN ANALYTIC THEOLOGY

Series Editors
Michael C. Rea   Oliver D. Crisp

OXFORD STUDIES IN ANALYTIC THEOLOGY

Analytic Theology utilizes the tools and methods of contemporary analytic philosophy for the purposes of constructive Christian theology, paying attention to the Christian tradition and development of doctrine. This innovative series of studies showcases high quality, cutting-edge research in this area, in monographs and symposia.

Analytic Christology and the Theological Interpretation of the New Testament

THOMAS H. MCCALL

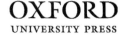

OXFORD
UNIVERSITY PRESS

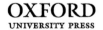

UNIVERSITY PRESS

Great Clarendon Street, Oxford, OX2 6DP,
United Kingdom

Oxford University Press is a department of the University of Oxford.
It furthers the University's objective of excellence in research, scholarship,
and education by publishing worldwide. Oxford is a registered trade mark of
Oxford University Press in the UK and in certain other countries

Published in the United States of America by Oxford University Press
198 Madison Avenue, New York, NY 10016, United States of America

British Library Cataloguing in Publication Data

Data available

Library of Congress Control Number: 2020945738

ISBN 978-0-19-885749-5

DOI: 10.1093/oso/9780198857495.001.0001

Printed and bound in the UK by
TJ Books Limited

Links to third party websites are provided by Oxford in good faith and
for information only. Oxford disclaims any responsibility for the materials
contained in any third party website referenced in this work.

For Alan Torrance

Acknowledgments

I am convinced that the project of constructive Christology has much to gain from deeper engagement with analytic theology and philosophy of religion. I am also convinced that the project of constructive Christology should be properly attuned to, and informed by, the insights of New Testament scholarship. In addition, I am convinced that there are points at which both analytic theology and biblical scholarship might benefit from inter-action with one another. This book is born out of those convictions. Accordingly, I employ the resources of both biblical scholarship and analytic Christology to make progress on some important issues in dogmatic Christology.

Various elements of some chapters have been previously published. Part of Chapter 1 can be found in the *Journal of Analytic Theology* (2020). Part of Chapter 4 was published in Caleb T. Friedeman, ed., *Listen, Understand, Obey: Essays in Honor of Gareth Lee Cockerill* (Eugene: Wipf and Stock, 2017). Part of Chapter 5 previously appeared as "Professor Ward and Polytheism," in *Philosophia Christi* (2016), and parts of Chapter 6 were published in the *Journal of Analytic Theology* (2019). These are published with the gracious permission of the editors.

I am well aware—in fact, *keenly* aware—of my own limitations in this effort. I am neither an analytic metaphysician nor a *Nuetestamentler*; I am merely a systematic theologian. Accordingly, I owe much to the great company of historical and systematic theologians, New Testament scholars, and analytic philosophers of religion who have done much to guide, inform, correct, and encourage me during this process. While of course all remain-ing errors and flaws are my own, I am especially indebted to the members of the Deerfield Dialogue Group: Doug Sweeney, Kevin J. Vanhoozer, James Arcadi, David Luy, Scott Manetsch, Dana Harris, Madison Pierce, Michelle Knight, Dick Averbeck, Lawson Younger, Eric Tully, and Steve Greggo. I am deeply grateful to members of the Logos Institute for Exegetical and Analytic Theology: Vi Bui, Harvey Cawdron, Joshua Cockayne, Kimberly Kroll, Jonathan Rutledge, Mitch Mallory, Tim Pawl, Faith Pawl, Preston Hill, Mike Rea, Oliver Crisp, Chandler Warren, Stephanie Nordby, Kevin Nordby, Koert Verhagen, Judith Wolfe, David Bennett, Stef McDade,

Katherine Scheussler, Sarah Shin, Christa McKirkland, Taylor Telford, and especially Andrew Torrance (with sincere apologies to any others who made helpful comments and criticisms but whose names I may have forgotten). The 2019–2020 Research Fellows of the Carl F. H. Henry Center for Theological Understanding (Paul Gould, Craig Bartholomew, Jordan Wessling, and Brian Matz, along with Matthew Wiley, Geoffrey Fulkerson, and Joel Chopp) read several chapters and gave helpful feedback. I also wish to express my gratitude to Jc Beall for his interest and very gracious encouragement: and to Douglas Campbell for his wonderfully spirited and invaluable interaction. Three anonymous referees for Oxford University Press offered extremely valuable suggestions and criticisms.

Alan Torrance has been a constant source of inspiration. I hope that this study is a proper (if inadequate) expression of gratitude, and truly it is an honor to dedicate this book to him.

Table of Contents

Introduction

Recent years have seen the flowering of something called the "theological interpretation of Scripture." This is, very roughly, what happens when biblical scholars and theologians alike read the Bible to see what it tells us about God. For several centuries, the discipline of biblical studies has been not only distinguished but also separated from theological discourse. There have been many notable exceptions, of course, but the all-too-common results have been these: biblical scholars often interpret the texts with other aims in mind (sometimes reading with a theological lens has been discouraged as unscholarly and thus improper), and theologians often do their work of constructive theology without serious engagement with biblical scholarship or even with the Christian Scriptures. Recent years have also seen the rise (or perhaps re-birth) of something now called "analytic theology." Analytic theology is, very roughly, what happens when philosophers who are interested in doctrine and theologians who think that there is (or might be) value in the appropriate use of philosophical tools get together. It is now a burgeoning movement, and analytic theologians are making contributions on a wide range of issues and topics, and from a variety of perspectives and approaches. We have not, however, witnessed a great deal of interaction between those who engage in the theological interpretation of Scripture and those who practice analytic theology.

In this work, I take a few steps toward bringing these two seemingly disparate approaches together. I do so out of the conviction that such an exercise might be beneficial for both disciplines. I do not see them as mutually exclusive; to the contrary, I am convinced that there is much room for conversation and that both might be better for it. I do so as a theologian, and I am keenly interested in a set of dogmatic questions and issues that have been and remain important. These are focused in Christology, and with respect to each of these questions or issues I work to make progress by marshaling the resources of both theological exegesis and analytic theology.

Analytic Christology and the Theological Interpretation of the New Testament. Thomas H. McCall, Oxford University Press (2021). © Thomas H. McCall. DOI: 10.1093/oso/9780198857495.003.0001

0.1 Analytic Theology and Reflection on Christ

Before proceeding further, it might be helpful to gain a bit more clarity on what is meant by terms such as "analytic theology" and "theological interpretation of the Bible" (or "theological exegesis"). Let us start with "analytic theology." We might simply consider analytic theology to be a way of doing systematic theology.[1] In this way of seeing things, it is, in William J. Abraham's words, "systematic theology attuned to the skills, resources, and virtues of analytic philosophy."[2] It is theology that is committed to clarity in expression and rigor in argument.[3] Seen this way, analytic theology is systematic theology done with a particular set of commitments, goals, and conceptual tools. Accordingly, analytic theology is simply theology done with a commitment to employ the resources of analytic philosophy where those conceptual tools might be helpful in the work of constructive Christian theology.[4]

Such a description may be helpful as an initial characterization, but it only takes us so far. The summary of Michael C. Rea takes us further, and it has become something of a standard account of analytic theology. Analytic theology is theology that shares much in common with the style and ambitions of analytic philosophy. As such, it is committed to the following desiderata:

(P1) Write as if philosophical positions and conclusions can be adequately formulated in sentences that can be formalized and logically manipulated;

(P2) Prioritize precision, clarity, and logical coherence;

(P3) Avoid substantive (non-decorative) use of metaphor and other tropes whose semantic content outstrips their propositional content;

(P4) Work as much as possible with well-understood primitive concepts, and concepts that can be analyzed in terms of those;

---

[1] As Oliver Crisp has recently argued, e.g. "Analytic Theology as Systematic Theology," *Journal of Open Theology* (2017), pp. 156–166.

[2] William J. Abraham, "Systematic Theology as Analytic Theology," in Oliver D. Crisp and Michael C. Rea, eds., *Analytic Theology: New Essays in the Philosophy of Theology* (Oxford: Oxford University Press, 2009), p. 54.

[3] See Oliver D. Crisp, "On Analytic Theology," in Oliver D. Crisp and Michael C. Rea, eds., *Analytic Theology: New Essays in the Philosophy of Theology* (Oxford: Oxford University Press, 2009), pp. 35–38.

[4] As I put it in *An Invitation to Analytic Christian Theology* (Downers Grove: InterVarsity Academic, 2015), p. 16.

(P5) Treat conceptual analysis (insofar as possible) as a source of evidence.[5]

We might usefully draw something of a distinction—albeit a rather rough and ready one—between what might be called "soft analytic theology" and "hard analytic theology." Soft analytic theology is simply any theology done with a commitment to the goals of clarity of expression, transparency and rigor of argument, and accountability with respect to broader intellectual standards. Hard analytic theology, on the other hand, does not hesitate to employ specific theories, arguments, or conclusions drawn from mainstream analytic epistemology, logic, metaphysics, esthetics, or moral theory. Hard analytic theology goes beyond its softer versions, for it takes actual work in analytic philosophy and presses it into service for the sake of doctrinal analysis and formulation. For instance, in analytic theological treatments of the doctrine of original sin, "soft" analytic theology strives for clarity of exposition and transparency and rigor of argument, while "hard" analytic theology may use recent developments in four-dimensionalist metaphysics in an effort to make sense of "realist" versions of the doctrine.[6] There is a sense in which the "soft" version should not even be controversial but should characterize all theology (although, sadly, it does not). But the "hard" cousin is sometimes rather more controversial and a bit more elusive; it is often less accessible to mainstream theologians and sometimes less interesting to them.[7]

0.2 Theological Interpretation and the Biblical Witness to Christ

What do I mean by "theological exegesis" and the "theological interpretation of Scripture?"

---

[5] Michael C. Rea, "Introduction," in Oliver D. Crisp and Michael C. Rea, eds., *Analytic Theology: New Essays on the Philosophy of Theology* (Oxford: Oxford University Press, 2009), pp. 5–6. For further discussion, see Thomas H. McCall, *An Introduction to Analytic Christian Theology* (Downers Grove: InterVarsity Academic, 2015), pp. 17–21.

[6] Thus a sterling example of "soft" analytic theology on the doctrine of original sin would be Ian McFarland, *In Adam's Fall: A Meditation on the Christian Doctrine of Original Sin* (Oxford: Wiley-Blackwell, 2010). To see excellent examples of "hard" analytic theology in action on this doctrine, see, e.g., Michael C. Rea, "The Metaphysics of Original Sin," in Peter van Inwagen and Dean Zimmerman, eds., *Persons: Human and Divine* (Oxford: Oxford University Press, 2007), pp. 319–356, and Hud Hudson, "Fission, Freedom, and the Fall," in Jonathan Kvanvig, ed., *Oxford Studies in Philosophy of Religion* (Oxford: Oxford University Press, 2009), pp. 58–79.

[7] Although perhaps *more* interesting to scholars who approach analytic theology as *philosophers*.

0.2.1 Theological Interpretation: An Initial Characterization

I mean something rather more than the characterization of Bruce L. McCormack when he says that "rightly understood, 'theological exegesis' is nothing more than the exegesis of passages whose content is theological."[8] I do not mean less than this, but I do mean something more. As John Webster puts it, "theological interpretation reads the New Testament as apostolic Scripture," and "it approaches the texts as acts of communication whose primary author is God the Holy Spirit acting in, with, and through the apostles."[9] To employ Daniel J. Treier's helpful summary, "theological exegesis deals with the Bible as a word about God and from God."[10] Accordingly, "Christians read the Bible as Scripture, authoritative as God's word for faith and life; thus, to interpret Scripture was to encounter God."[11] Beyond this, there are several points that are important for a proper understanding of theological interpretation (as I see it, at least). First, while theological interpretation need not be opposed to historical-critical study of the Bible and indeed stands to benefit from it (and especially from the wealth of knowledge offered by experts in studies of the ancient Near East, Second Temple Judaism, and relevant Greco-Roman contexts), theological interpretation is neither reducible to such study nor even finally accountable to conformity to the conclusions of such studies.[12] Second, theological interpretation views traditional (including "pre-critical") exegesis as a potential source of insight and such exegetes as fellow sojourners, allies,

[8] Bruce L. McCormack, "The Identity of the Son: Karl Barth's Exegesis of Hebrews 1.1-4 (and Similar Passages)," in Jon C. Laansma and Daniel J. Treier, eds., *Christology, Hermeneutics, and Hebrews: Profiles from the History of Interpretation* (New York: Bloomsbury T&T Clark, 2012), p. 158.
[9] John Webster, "One Who is Son: Theological Reflections on the Exordium to the Epistle to the Hebrews," in Richard Bauckham, Daniel R. Driver, Trevor A. Hart, and Nathan MacDonald, eds., *The Epistle to the Hebrews and Christian Theology* (Grand Rapids: William B. Eerdmans Publishing Co., 2009), p. 69.
[10] Daniel J. Treier, *Introducing Theological Interpretation of Scripture: Recovering a Christian Practice* (Grand Rapids: Baker Academic, 2008), p. 36.
[11] Treier, *Introducing Theological Interpretation*, p. 13.
[12] For the responsible theological exegete, there may be occasions when outright rejection of such conclusions is entirely warranted. See Peter van Inwagen, "Critical Studies of the New Testament and the User of the New Testament," in Thomas P. Flint and Eleonore Stump, eds., *Hermes and Athena: Biblical Exegesis and Philosophical Theology* (Notre Dame: University of Notre Dame Press, 1993), pp. 159–190; Alvin Plantinga, *Warranted Christian Belief* (Oxford: Oxford University Press, 2000), pp. 374–421; C. Stephen Evans, *The Historical Christ and the Jesus of Faith: The Incarnational Narrative as History* (Oxford: Oxford University Press, 1996).

and mentors.[13] This does not, of course, mean that some interpretation is better simply by virtue of being older (exegesis isn't fine wine, nor is it like it in all respects), nor does it mean that the responsible theological exegete must agree with all that has been said in the past (indeed, it is *impossible* to do so). But rather than assuming that whatever is most recent is obviously better than what came before, the proper approach is one of respect and humility. Third, while theological interpretation should not neglect historical-grammatical approaches, it proceeds with a conviction that proper inter-pretation of any particular text should be done within the broader *canonical* context. In a manner not dissimilar to the theories of "emergence" that are popular in the philosophy of physics and the philosophy of biology, the whole has properties that are not reducible to the sum of the parts, and it is not possible to arrive at a fulsome and adequate understanding of those parts without appreciation both for those "emergent" properties and for the kind of "top-down" causal effect that they have. Fourth, and more controversially, theological exegesis (again, as I am doing it here) is disposed to view creedal formulations as aids to proper exegesis rather than as barriers to the proper understanding of Scripture. C. Kavin Rowe is correct when he says that there is an "organic connection between the biblical testimony and the early creeds, and the creeds can serve as hermeneutical guidelines to reading the Bible because it is the biblical text itself that necessitated the credal formulations."[14]

0.3 A Preview of Coming Attractions

The proof is, according to the old cliché, in the pudding. So perhaps it will help to offer an overview of what follows. I begin with chapters that offer analytic engagement with important issues and recent proposals in New Testament studies. In Chapter 1, I take a close look at Paul's claims to be "crucified" with Christ and to now share life with the incarnate Son. Engaging especially with "apocalyptic" interpretations of Paul, I offer theo-logical analysis of the current discussion, look at how the current debate in biblical scholarship might map onto various metaphysical options, and propose a way forward. In Chapter 2, I offer an analysis of the debate over

---

[13] The *locus classicus* of the recent revival is David C. Steinmetz, "The Superiority of Pre-Critical Exegesis," *Theology Today* (1980), pp. 27–38.

[14] C. Kavin Rowe, "Luke and the Trinity: An Essay in Ecclesial Biblical Theology," *Scottish Journal of Theology* (2003), p. 4.

the "faith of Christ" in contemporary New Testament scholarship. Here I take stock of the major extant proposals, and I suggest that theological analysis shows that retrieval of older interpretations can help us adjudicate this debate and move forward constructively.

In Chapter 3, I turn to consideration of some important issues in dogmatic Christology as these are treated by "systematic" theologians, and I bring both exegetical and analytic resources to bear upon contemporary debates. Here I bring attention to the identity of the Son. Recent debates over whether we can and should think of Christ as the *logos asarkos* are the focus here. Contemporary debates over the proper interpretation of the theology of Karl Barth have spawned additional interesting debates about Christology and theology proper, and these are the subject of this chapter. Accordingly, I first outline Bruce L. McCormack's controversial interpretive proposal about the relation of the doctrine of election to Christology and the doctrine of the Trinity in Barth's mature doctrine of God; following this I offer an account of McCormack's own constructive proposal. I then survey the theological criticisms that are brought against it; here I look not only at the criticisms that are raised with respect to the proper interpretation of Barth but also and primarily at the crucial doctrinal issues. This leads to a theological analysis of the proposal. Remaining in conversation with Barth, Chapter 4 addresses the nature of the Son's obedience or submission. Proceeding in direct conversation with the proposals of Karl Barth and Thomas Aquinas, I first summarize their positions, then raise some important theological issues, and then ask what a properly theological interpretation of Hebrews 5:8 contributes to the discussion.

In Chapter 5, I turn to exegetically driven theological analysis of recent proposals made by analytic theologians and philosophers of religion. I turn attention to the important issue of the relation of the Son to the Father. I approach this issue by first surveying some of the recent debates over "social" doctrines of the Trinity. I work to gain some clarity on what is (or might be) meant by the term "Social Trinity" as a label, I engage with theological exegesis of some important New Testament texts that are directly relevant to the contemporary discussions, and I apply this work to an analysis of the recent analytic Trinitarian theology of Keith Ward. Finally, in Chapter 6, I offer engagement with Jc Beall's bold and novel suggestion that we accept the traditional doctrine of the incarnation as a genuine contradiction. Here I raise some distinctly theological concerns; in addition to several issues that are historically grounded, I raise some concerns for his view that come directly from the theological interpretation of the New Testament witness to Christ.

1

Crucified with Christ

The *Ego* and the *Omega*

1.1 Introduction

Paul's declaration at the conclusion of the second chapter of his letter to the
Galatians is arresting. It is also rather unsettling, and it raises some very
interesting exegetical and important theological issues.[1] After saying that
those persons (and here he uses Ἡμεῖς to include himself) who are of Jewish
ethnicity know that they are "justified" not through the works of the law but
by faith in Christ, after testifying that "we too have put our faith in Christ
Jesus that we may be justified by faith in Christ" (Gal 2:15–16), and after
adamantly denying that justification through such faith somehow legitim-
izes sin (μή γένοιτο), Paul makes this statement:

> For through the law I died to the law so that I might live for God. I have
> been crucified with Christ and I no longer live, but Christ lives in me. The
> life I live in the body (ἐν σαρχί), I live by faith in the Son of God, who loved
> me and gave himself for me (Gal 2:19–20).

Strikingly, Paul claims that "I am crucified with Christ" and "I no longer live,
but Christ lives in me." What does he mean? Grant Macaskill says that this
text is "suggestive of an absolute transformation of identity."[2] But just who is
this "I" who no longer lives? Who is the "I" who is said to now live? What is

---

[1] This passage is challenging at several levels (including exegesis). As N. T. Wright says, these
are "deliberately rich and dense formulations," *Paul and His Recent Interpreters: Some
Contemporary Debates* (Minneapolis: Fortress Press, 2015), p. 105. It is also central to Paul's
theology. To quote Wright again, he says that this is the "decisive climax" of Paul's teaching,
Paul and His Recent Interpreters, pp. 342–343. Martinus C. de Boer concurs: this is "the
theological high point of the first two chapters," *Galatians: A Commentary* (Louisville:
Westminster John Knox Press, 2011), p. 159.

[2] Grant Macaskill, *Union with Christ in the New Testament* (Oxford: Oxford University
Press, 2013), p. 221, cf., p. 225.

Analytic Christology and the Theological Interpretation of the New Testament. Thomas H. McCall,
Oxford University Press (2021). © Thomas H. McCall. DOI: 10.1093/oso/9780198857495.003.0002

the relation of these "I"s to one another? And how are the themes of union with Christ—and, indeed, participation in Christ—to be understood? Indeed, is the right account of the relation of the "I" to Christ somehow even stronger than what can be captured by language of "union" and "participation?" Is it identity?

In this essay I offer a closer look at this text and some of the issues raised by it. I do so as a sort of analytic intervention into a debate among the so-called "apocalyptic" interpreters of Paul. Apocalyptic exegetes offer engagement with Paul's writings that is refreshingly and overtly theological. Their exegesis is often insightful and theologically fecund, and it holds significant promise for theology done in dogmatic and analytic modes. Gratefully engaging with apocalyptic interpretations, my aim throughout is to work toward a better understanding of Paul's account of these matters.[3] Accordingly, I begin by comparing the interpretations offered by what I refer to as the "Modest Apocalyptic" (MA) and "Radical Apocalyptic" (RA) interpretations of the text. I then offer some analysis of these claims and their entailments, and I raise some theological concerns about the RA proposals. I then revisit a traditional reading with an eye toward the possibilities of *ressourcement* and conclude with a modest proposal that takes insights from both traditional and apocalyptic approaches.

1.2 The Apocalyptic Interpretations of Paul

1.2.1 The Apocalyptic Paul

So-called "Apocalyptic" interpretations of Paul have seen great gains in popularity and influence (within scholarly circles) over the course of the past few decades. Such interpretations differ sharply from older "Protestant" or "Lutheran" readings. But they also differ—and in some cases they differ very sharply—from more recent "New Perspectives" on Paul (NPP). For all their important differences, both the older "Lutheran" and NPP

---

[3] I am aware that this approach is atypical among scholars of Pauline theology, which tends to be, as Macaskill has pointed out, "largely concerned with divine *action* and not with categories of *nature* or *being...*" However, as Macaskill also recognizes and argues, it is very difficult to make adequate sense of Paul's theology without due attention to the broader issues related to metaphysics and ontology. Grant Macaskill, "Dynamic Reciprocity and Ontological Affinity in the Pauline Account of Solidarity," *International Journal of Systematic Theology* 22:1 (2020), pp. 18–28 (here p. 19).

interpretations share a basic and fundamental understanding of strong continuity between the "old" that has become soiled and poisoned and ruined by sin and the "new" that is revealed and inaugurated in Christ. The big story, as told by both traditional Protestant interpreters and the proponents of the NPP, strongly emphasizes the place and prominence of *covenant* within that story. Traditional and NPP interpreters commonly insist that what was marred and broken and ruined by sin is reclaimed and repaired and reconciled by God's decisive action in the work of Jesus Christ. Traditional theologians and the advocates of the NPP have serious disagreements among themselves about important issues within that broad understanding. Famously, the older "Lutheran" readings see Jewish "legalism" and the accompanying efforts to somehow merit or earn salvation through good works as the culprit, while the proponents of the NPP typically aver that the older theologies rest upon misunderstandings of Second Temple Judaism and instead insist that Jewish thought was committed to "covenantal nomism." But despite such disagreements—however serious and sharp they may be—there is a general sense of shared agreement that what God is doing in Christ maintains important continuity with the covenant that God made with Israel for the sake of the world.

Apocalyptic interpretations of Paul question—and often reject—this basic assumption of continuity. Instead, apocalyptic readings of Paul insist that the gospel is an in-breaking that disrupts all that came before. Apocalyptic theologians insist that the "full scope, depth, and radicality of the gospel of God" demands that we account for the "actual and manifest contradiction of that gospel" by the world.[4] This world, the world as it is—indeed, "*the* world" in Pauline usage of the term—is something that has been taken over and is now controlled by sin. As J. Louis Martyn puts it, "we would not be totally wrong to say – with the poetic language of tragedy – that Sin is virtually the *creator* of *this* world."[5] This world, as it is, is something that is "not under the immediate and exclusive hegemony either of God or of human beings"; instead, it is under the control of evil powers and is thus "the frightening, horrifying scene of genuine and profound disaster."[6] In direct response to this disaster, God has acted decisively—indeed, *apocalyptically*—in Christ.

---

[4] Philip G. Ziegler, *Militant Grace: The Apocalyptic Turn and the Future of Christian Theology* (Grand Rapids: Baker Academic, 2018), p. 26.

[5] J. Louis Martyn, "World Without End or Twice-Invaded World," in Christine Roy Yoder, et al., eds., *Shaking Heaven and Earth: Essays in Honor of Walter Brueggemann and Charles B. Cousar* (Louisville: Westminster John Knox Press, 2005), p. 120.

[6] Martyn, "World Without End," p. 122.

God's work in Christ is a truly radical invasion. In Christ, God "is not merely repairing *this* world" but instead is creating a completely new one that is "in fundamental contrast to *this* world."[7] Such a radical rupture means that God's revelation in Christ is a "break with the ultimate authority of the Torah," as John M. G. Barclay puts it, for "the cross of Christ shatters every ordered system of norms, however embedded in the seemingly 'natural' order of 'the world.' "[8]

All genuine knowledge of God is disclosed in Christ.[9] Indeed, for some very influential proponents of apocalyptic Pauline theology, any claims to knowledge of God that do not both begin and terminate in Christ are to be held at arm's length. The worry here is that such claims are not only mistaken but indeed idolatrous. In other words, any claims to knowledge of God via "natural theology" are both false and dangerous. Douglas A. Campbell, for instance, energetically polemicizes against what he refers to as "Justification Theory." As he sees things, Justification Theory has exerted massive influence in the history of Christian theology. The term "justification" seems to be doing double duty for Campbell here, for he uses it in reference to epistemology as well as soteriology. Epistemologically, Justification Theory relies upon a kind of foundationalism according to which both the basic (or "foundational") facts about God and sin are known through natural theology (along the lines of what Campbell takes to be the all-too-common misreading of Rom 1:18–32). From "nature" we are to learn that God exists and that humans are responsible and legally or forensically guilty before God for their sins; we learn about the problem from natural theology, and the gospel is the solution to that problem. Campbell protests against this approach, and he insists as well that the legal account of salvation ("justification" in the soteriological sense) is skewed from the outset. Campbell resists such an approach as overly individualistic and "contractualist" (as well as foundationalist).[10] Campbell reads the opening chapters of Romans (and similar passages scattered elsewhere in the Pauline corpus) as "speech-in-character" that actually articulate the views of the *opponents* of the gospel, and he mounts an

---

[7] Martyn, "World Without End," p. 126.

[8] John M. G. Barclay, *Paul and the Gift* (Grand Rapids: William B. Eerdmans Publishing Co., 2015), p. 394. He continues: "All other criteria of value have been discounted by their superordinate worth of belonging to Christ," p. 429.

[9] See the discussion in Ziegler, *Militant Grace*, p. 27.

[10] The terms "individualist" and "contractualist" feature prominently in Joshua W. Jipp's overview of Campbell's work. See Joshua W. Jipp, "Douglas Campbell's Apocalyptic, Rhetorical Paul: Review Article," *Horizons in Biblical Theology* 32:2 (2010), pp. 183–197.

extended and very vigorous argument that the true gospel is radically opposed to such notions. Where the older readings (either Roman Catholic or Protestant, and whether "old" or "new" perspective) saw the gospel as the solution to a problem that was revealed and understood prior to the in-breaking of God's gospel in Christ, Campbell's genuinely apocalyptic reading will have none of that. Where the older views took the gospel to be about the legal status of individuals who had done bad things, Campbell's account proclaims good news that is communitarian and participatory. And where the older doctrines maintain that some part of a God-human contract must be fulfilled or completed from the human side (either in perfect obedience to the law or in the exercise of *faith*), Campbell insists that the authentic gospel rejects all such contractual arrangements in favor of genuine grace that is *covenantal* and thus non-conditional. The upshot of this should be clear (or, at least, clear enough for present purposes): Paul's gospel is radical and radically apocalyptic. It upends all prior conceptions of what God—and, indeed, all proper concepts of everything else in relation to God—is really like. It confounds all worldly wisdom. It abolishes any idolatrous notions about the adequacy of human agency. And it demonstrates the finality of God's authentic revelation in Christ. The gospel is something that is *new*, and it proclaims a *new creation*, a *new life* that is *in Christ*.

Of course, not all exegetes and theologians associated with the "apocalyptic school" would agree with Campbell on all these points, and many New Testament scholars have deep and fundamental disagreements with his proposal. Francis Watson, for instance, resists being lumped in with the proponents of "Justification Theory" (at least as Campbell depicts it), but he also rejects Campbell's proposal as "neo-Marcionite."[11] Campbell's unrelenting insistence on the radical in-breaking and utterly disruptive nature of God's revelation in Christ is, however, reflective of something that is widespread and important within apocalyptic theology.

---

[11] Francis Watson, *Paul and the Hermeneutics of Faith*, second edition (New York: Bloomsbury T&T Clark, 2016), p. xlv. Watson says that Campbell's *Deliverance* is a work of "perverse brilliance." Barclay says that Campbell sounds "most like Marcion" and is "strongly reminiscent of Marcion," *Paul and the Gift*, pp. 173, 465 n41. R. Barry Matlock judges Campbell's account of Justification Theory to be "the most elaborately constructed straw man [he] has ever witnessed, and to watch Campbell parry and thrust with it across hundreds of sprawling pages is a singular and uncanny spectacle," and he says that Campbell's accusations against it "alternate between calumny and farce," R. Barry Matlock, "Zeal for Paul but Not According to Knowledge: Douglas Campbell's War on 'Justification Theory,'" *Journal for the Study of the New Testament* 34:2 (2011), p. 137.

With this brief background in mind, let us now turn to the exegesis of Gal 2:19–20. Some of the leading apocalyptic interpreters seem rather unsure of what to make of the striking claims made by Paul in Gal 2:19–20. Not surprisingly, they generally are not attracted to the older and more traditional interpretations, but some are hesitant to endorse a more thoroughgoing or even "literal" understanding of Paul's claims. Thus Martyn takes Paul to be using the verb in a "nonliteral manner."[12] Paul is, he says, not merely a follower or disciple of Jesus but someone who is co-crucified, but Paul's claim is to be understood in something less than a literal sense. The "main accent" of Paul's statement "'to be 'crucified with Christ' lies, therefore, on incorporation into the Christ whose own path determines the destiny of those who are bound to him."[13] Martinus C. de Boer is struck by the force of Paul's "extreme language of crucifixion with Christ."[14] But he says that Paul's claims "cannot be taken literally," for while this is "realistic and serious" (cf. 5:24; 6:14), nonetheless the "language is metaphorical and hyperbolic."[15] On his view, "to 'die to something' is metaphorical and means to be separated from it" (cf. Rom 6:2, 10, 11; 7:6). And in this case, "Paul's 'I' (*ego*) has ceased to exist" *in reference to its orientation to the law*; what is gone is not the person known as Paul but instead the "nomistic 'I' – the 'I' that finds its identity and its hope of justification (5:5) in (the observance of) the law – that has died."[16] It is the "nomistically determined 'I'" who is gone, the "'I' that was a zealot for the ancestral traditions and persecuted God's church" (1:13–14).[17] In place of this old "I" is the "new identity, a new self" that is delighted and energetic in the apostolic proclamation of the singularity and finality of the gospel of Jesus Christ.[18]

Let us refer to these readings as "Modest-Apocalyptic" interpretations. But other apocalyptic interpreters are not satisfied with such readings.

1.2.2 Radical Apocalyptic Options

Some of the claims made by apocalyptic interpreters suggest much more radical readings of Paul's claim. We will, then, call these "Radical-Apocalyptic" readings. Drawing upon a particular reading of Martin Luther's

---

[12] James Louis Martyn, *Galatians: A New Translation and Commentary* (New Haven: Yale University Press, 1997), p. 278.
[13] Martyn, *Galatians*, p. 279. [14] de Boer, *Galatians*, p. 161.
[15] de Boer, *Galatians*, p. 160. [16] de Boer, *Galatians*, p. 159.
[17] de Boer, *Galatians*, p. 161. [18] de Boer, *Galatians*, p. 161.

theology, Stephen Chester says that for the Reformer, union with Christ "does not work on the basis of a transformation of the self of the Christian. It works rather on the basis of the leaving behind and abandoning of that self."[19] To speak of a "changed or renewed life is therefore potentially misleading," because the central point concerns the "re-creation of the person."[20] Beverly Roberts Gaventa forcefully emphasizes the discontinuity between the old and the new. She insists upon the "singularity" of the gospel of Christ; by this she means not only the fact that there is only one gospel (cf. Gal 1:6-9) but also "its singular, all-encompassing action in the lives of human beings."[21] The gospel—the one and only true gospel, *the* gospel of Jesus Christ—"claims all that a human is; the gospel becomes the locus of human identity; the gospel replaces the old cosmos."[22] When we come to the "radical and radically troubling" message that is encapsulated in Paul's claim about co-crucifixion, we are taken into the "heart" of Paul's "understanding of the gospel."[23] Paul's claim is not merely that Christ is teacher or example, nor is it even that Jesus is Lord.[24] Rather, it is that he is *crucified with* the Christ who is teacher and Lord; he shares in Christ's brutal execution as Christ bears the full weight and force of evil and sin.

Gaventa protests against the moves made by de Boer. For in this context, she exclaims, "there is no sign that this death and life are the death and life of the nomistic self only (although that is included)."[25] No indeed. It is nothing less than "the whole of the ἐγώ that is gone."[26] Gaventa follows Campbell when he says that Paul is "speaking of the execution of his own identity, and his immersion in Christ's."[27] Gaventa understands "that there is still life in a human body, of course."[28] But she also insists that "by moving to the

---

[19] Stephen Chester, "Apocalyptic Union: Martin Luther's Account of Faith in Christ," in Michael J. Thate, Kevin J. Vanhoozer, Constantine R. Campbell, eds., *"In Christ" in Paul: Explorations of Paul's Theology of Union and Participation* (Grand Rapids: William B. Eerdmans Publishing Co., 2018), p. 386.

[20] Chester, "Apocalyptic Union," p. 386.

[21] Beverly Roberts Gaventa, "The Singularity of the Gospel Revisited," in Mark W. Elliott, Scott J. Hafemann, N. T. Wright, and John Frederick, eds., *Galatians and Christian Theology: Justification, the Gospel, and Ethics in Paul's Letter* (Grand Rapids: Baker Academic, 2014), p. 188.

[22] Gaventa, "The Singularity of the Gospel Revisited," p. 188.

[23] Gaventa, "The Singularity of the Gospel Revisited," pp. 188, 193.

[24] Gaventa, "The Singularity of the Gospel Revisited," p. 193.

[25] Gaventa, "The Singularity of the Gospel Revisited," p. 193.

[26] Gaventa, "The Singularity of the Gospel Revisited," p. 193.

[27] Douglas Campbell, *The Deliverance of God: An Apocalyptic Rereading of Justification in Paul* (Grand Rapids: William B. Eerdmans Publishing Co., 2009), p. 848. She does not note that Campbell adds that Paul "is still distinguishable as a person within this process."

[28] Gaventa, "The Singularity of the Gospel Revisited," p. 194.

language of 'death' and 'life,' Paul has again shifted his discourse."[29] The gospel is not only about legality, for the "canvas on which Paul depicts the gospel has enlarged from legal language to existential language."[30] The gospel is not merely about justification or "rectification"—instead, "from Paul's perspective," it is "singular in that it is all-consuming: there is no more ἐγώ."[31]

Gaventa is not alone. Paul Nadim Tarzi insists that the radical change is no "mere psychological shift," and he insists that "our 'I' – that is, our very self – does not live anymore, It is truly dead," and "Pauline terminology fully equates life with Christ."[32] John M. G. Barclay makes similar claims. As Gaventa notes, he says that "Paul refers to the real and total demolition of the self, as previously constituted."[33] Barclay is certain that the crucifixion marks a "radical disjunction" with what has come before.[34] Paul's statement about Christ living "in" him "gestures to the resurrection (1:1), which founds a radically new existence."[35] Barclay goes on to say that out of the newness of this resurrected Christ-life, "every value is newly evaluated and every norm reassessed."[36] Beyond this, however, he goes on to say that "Paul depicts the believer's agency as both replaced ('It is no longer I who live...') and remade ('the life I now live...')."[37] He argues that "Paul uses multiple expressions to indicate the creation, in baptism, of a new subjectivity generated by, and dependent on, the Christ-event: believers are 'baptized into Christ,' have 'put on Christ,' constitute one person 'in Christ,' and henceforth 'belong to Christ'" (3:27–29).[38] Notice the strength of the claims: not only is there a "new subjectivity" (that apparently is singular), but those who are baptized "into Christ" are said to "constitute one person." Barclay recognizes that his reading of Gal 2:20 (along with 3:27–29 and 4:19) "complicates notions of agency in Pauline thought."[39] The agency of those who belong to Christ and are "in Christ" "is by no means self-generated or independent, let alone autonomous."[40] "At the same time," as Barclay notes, "Paul has no hesitation in speaking of believers as agents."[41] The result of

[29]   Gaventa, "The Singularity of the Gospel Revisited," p. 194.
[30]   Gaventa, "The Singularity of the Gospel Revisited," p. 194.
[31]   Gaventa, "The Singularity of the Gospel Revisited," p. 195.
[32]   Paul Nadim Tarzi, *Galatians: A Commentary* (Crestwood, NY: St. Vladimir's Seminary Press, 1994), p. 89.
[33]   John M. G. Barclay, "Paul's Story: Theology as Testimony," in Bruce W. Longenecker, ed., *Narrative Dynamics in Paul: A Critical Assessment* (Louisville: Westminster John Knox, 2002), p. 143, cited in Gaventa, "The Singularity of the Gospel Revisited," p. 193 n22.
[34]   Barclay, *Paul and the Gift*, p. 386.   [35]   Barclay, *Paul and the Gift*, p. 386.
[36]   Barclay, *Paul and the Gift*, p. 386.   [37]   Barclay, *Paul and the Gift*, p. 386.
[38]   Barclay, *Paul and the Gift*, p. 396.   [39]   Barclay, *Paul and the Gift*, p. 441.
[40]   Barclay, *Paul and the Gift*, p. 441.   [41]   Barclay, *Paul and the Gift*, p. 441.

co-crucifixion is not only a network of "new social relations" but indeed "the reconstitution of each individual self (Gal 2:19–20)."[42]

Taking a position similar to that of Gaventa, Jonathan Linebaugh resists the strategy offered by de Boer. It cannot be the case that it is merely the "nomistically determined 'I'" who is put to death with Christ, and to read Paul's statement as "metaphorical and hyperbolic" is to miss Paul's main point. Indeed, Linebaugh claims that "it is just this assumption" (that the claim should be read metaphorically rather than literally) that "Paul's confession resists."[43] For "Galatians 2:20 is not an analogy between Christ's death and a death-like experience of the I. Galatians 2:20, rather, is an announcement that Christ's death is the death of the I. To retreat to the language of non-literal and hyperbolic is to miss the radical reframing required by Paul's language."[44] Linebaugh refuses to accept any easy "domestication" of Paul's "confession of death."[45] He is especially concerned to resist the temptation offered by traditional interpreters such as Aquinas. As Linebaugh reads him, what dies on Aquinas's interpretation is not the *person* but the inclination to sin that corrupts the person. Aquinas's maxim that *gratia non tollit naturam sed perficit* ("grace does not destroy but perfects nature") means that the "new creature" is "not so much new as renewed" and that "the 'I', in other words, survives their salvation."[46] Against traditional interpretations such as those of Aquinas, Linebaugh closely links "God's unconditioned grace" in "three radical forms: *creatio ex nihilo, resurrectio moruorum*, and *iustificatio impii*."[47] He links these together to form a "confession of *creatio ex nihilo* in the language of salvation *sola gratia*: 'out of nothing' means 'by grace alone...'"[48] The one who is justified is thus "constituted as 'a new creature,'" and this new creation is something that happens "*ex nihilo*."[49]

Linebaugh is, however, bothered by a worry that is raised by Daphne Hampson. Hampson is concerned that an account of strict identity with Christ would result in the evaporation of the "I." If the believer and Christ are really "one person," then does not the "otherness" of the "I" in the "I-Thou" relationship collapse? And if there is no "I," then how could there

[42] Barclay, *Paul and the Gift*, p. 568.
[43] Jonathan Linebaugh, "The Speech of the Dead: Identifying the No Longer and the Now Living 'I' of Galatians 2:20," *New Testament Studies* 66:1 (2019), p. 92.
[44] Linebaugh, "The Speech of the Dead," p. 92.
[45] Linebaugh, "The Speech of the Dead," p. 94.
[46] Linebaugh, "The Speech of the Dead," p. 94.
[47] Linebaugh, "The Speech of the Dead," p. 97.
[48] Linebaugh, "The Speech of the Dead," p. 97.
[49] Linebaugh, "The Speech of the Dead," p. 98.

be an "I" to give or receive love? If "the self does not survive salvation," then what—and *who*—are we talking about?[50] Who is doing the talking? And what sense can we make of "saving" something or someone that does not survive? Linebaugh wrestles with this worry: "Does the announcement of the death of the I eliminate the possibility of God's love for the I? If I am only outside myself and in Christ, does God ever look at and love me?"[51] So is there continuity between the "no longer living and the now living I?"[52] Linebaugh is deeply skeptical of any attempts to ground the continuity in creation or "nature"; he remains stoutly opposed to Aquinas's view. As we have seen, he has little patience for the hesitations of Martyn and de Boer, and certainly there is no possibility of going back to the older views. But he also sees the need to maintain some genuine continuity between the "I" that is in Christ and the "I" that preceded it. He finally opts for the view that "Paul's 'strange and un-heard of' confession requires a dialectical conclusion..."[53] So on one hand, the answer is a clear and unambiguous "No: death and life divide the no longer and the now living I and the life of the latter is gifted, ex-centric, and in Christ."[54] But on the other hand, the answer is an unequivocal and emphatic "Yes: though I no longer live, there is a me that is ever and always loved."[55] For while it is true that "the human self cannot, at least not self-referentially, be said to survive its own salvation," yet it is also said to somehow be true that this does not mean that there is "no self that is in some sense the same self before and after the cross."[56]

1.3 Toward Theological Analysis

D. H. Bertschmann observes that such a radical "notion of grace, while teeming with hope and wonder, also generates questions."[57] She especially

---

[50] Linebaugh, "The Speech of the Dead," p. 103.
[51] Linebaugh, "The Speech of the Dead," p. 103.
[52] Linebaugh, "The Speech of the Dead," p. 104.
[53] Linebaugh, "The Speech of the Dead," p. 105.
[54] Linebaugh, "The Speech of the Dead," p. 105.
[55] Linebaugh, "The Speech of the Dead," p. 105.
[56] Jonathan A. Linebaugh, "Incongruous and Creative Grace: Reading *Paul and the Gift* with Martin Luther," *International Journal of Systematic Theology* 22:1 (2020), p. 58. I take the "in some sense" seriously here. Without it, we are left with what appears to be a straightforward contradiction—and thus a necessary falsehood. But the "in some sense" cries out for some explanation.
[57] D. H. Bertschmann, "*Ex Nihilo* or *Tabula Rasa*? God's Grace between Freedom and Fidelity," *International Journal of Systematic Theology* 22:1 (2020), p. 32.

wants to know what we make of the claims about divine creation out of nothing: "if God creates individuals and people anew in an act of *creatio ex nihilo*, what happens to the old creations of both individuals and communities?"[58]

1.3.1 Replacement Theories

Some of the apocalyptic proposals seem to be saying nothing less than this: the person or the "I" is actually destroyed or demolished but then a new person is made in place of the old. Some expressions of the RA approach seem to be saying this but then also going on to claim that there indeed *is* also *some* continuity between the "old I" and the "new I." So there both is and is not continuity between "them." Despite appearances, perhaps these claims are not—at least in all cases—intended as claims about the sober metaphysical truth.[59] But they surely *seem* to be making such claims, and what they say is, minimally, at least suggestive of a such claims. So what are we to make of them?

Some statements made by these theological interpreters would seem to suggest that the individual or self or "I"—presumably the *person*—is annihilated but then somehow replaced. As we have seen, theological interpreters of Pauline theology claim that:

- "the whole of the ἐγώ is gone" and "there is no more ἐγώ" (Gaventa);
- Paul is "speaking of the execution of his own identity" (Campbell);
- "Paul refers to the real and total demolition of the self" (Barclay);
- "the believer's agency is both replaced...and remade" as a "new subjectivity" that is "the reconstitution of each individual self" (Barclay); and
- one who is joined in union with Christ is "constituted as 'a new creature'" who is "made *ex nihilo*" (Linebaugh).

---

[58] Bertschmann, "*Ex Nihilo* or *Tabula Rasa*," p. 32.
[59] Despite Linebaugh's forceful protest against what he recalls a "retreat" to "non-literal" understandings, it is less than obvious that even he can really take the language *literally*. After all, surely he thinks that the crucifixion of Christ was an actual historical event in which the physical body of Jesus was nailed to a wooden cross—but presumably he does not think that this is also true of either Paul or other believers (including, presumably, himself), Linebaugh, "The Speech of the Dead," p. 92.

Taken straightforwardly, we might conclude from such statements that the proper meaning of Paul's teaching includes these elements: first, the self or "I" or person is demolished or annihilated; second, that the annihilated person is replaced with a new creation that bears strong similarities to the former one; and, third, that, despite such similarities, there is no continuity of personal identity between the old and the new, for there is no "I" who "survives their salvation."[60]

It is not immediately obvious just what to make of these claims. Consider again Linebaugh's appeal to the doctrine of *creatio ex nihilo*, and recall that for him, anything "less" (anything that would allow the human nature to be merely "radically altered" and "perfected and healed" rather than destroyed and replaced) is a "domestication" of Paul's doctrine.[61] Taking this seriously, we might opt for something like an occasionalist account of the position.[62] Speaking strictly and "literally," the first Paul (call it P1) is something that passes from existence and then is replaced by another Paul (call it P2) in a moment of re-creation. This creation is an act that is *ex nihilo*. Of course, this would not be plausible as an instance of a general or what we could call "global" account of occasionalism. For if occasionalism is true as a general or global account, then, at least on common or standard accounts of what occasionalism is, then there would be nothing special (in this sense, at least) about the event of co-crucifixion. For if we accept occasionalism as an overall account of creation and providence, then the world and every (created) entity in it is being re-created out of nothing at every moment. So, if occasionalism were true as a general or global account of reality, then there would be nothing radical or apocalyptic or even unusual about the Christ-event and anyone's co-crucifixion relation to it. To the contrary, we would have business as usual: sure, Paul is being re-created out of nothing at the moment of his union with Christ in the crucifixion, but, on occasionalism, Paul is *always* being re-created out of nothing. And so is everyone and everything else.

So global occasionalism would not seem to be an attractive option, and in point of fact it might be bad news for the apocalyptic interpretations if occasionalism were true as a general or overall account of reality. But

---

[60] Linebaugh, "The Speech of the Dead," p. 104.

[61] Linebaugh, "The Speech of the Dead," p. 94.

[62] For a helpful account of occasionalism set within the late medieval and early modern contexts, see Alfred J. Freddoso, "Medieval Aristotelianism and the Case Against Secondary Causation in Nature," in Thomas V. Morris, ed., *Divine and Human Action: Essays in the Metaphysics of Theism* (Ithaca: Cornell University Press, 1988), pp. 74–118.

something *like* occasionalism, or what we might call "local occasionalism," might be the right way to go. On this proposal it is not the case that *everything* is being re-created at every moment, nor is it the case that *Paul* is continually being re-created out of nothing. But at one decisive moment— the moment of Paul's being joined in union with Christ—there is complete replacement of P1 with some divinely created P2. From here the metaphysical options open up. If one is a physicalist, then what is replaced by the de novo creation is Paul's body; the body that is P1 is replaced by the body that is P2.[63] If some version of hylomorphism is the right way to think about such matters, then what is replaced by the new creation is the particular body-soul composite that is—or was—Paul. If one is a proponent of broadly Lockean psychological continuity theories, then what is replaced is the stream of consciousness. If one holds out for "narrative self-constitution," then what changes is the story in which one is embedded and the context that shapes the identity.[64] If one is a mind-body dualist of more Cartesian commitments, then perhaps what is replaced is actually only the *soul* that is P1. Perhaps the body that happens to be inhabited by P1 remains the same, or maybe not. Either way, the important point is that the *real* P1—whatever exactly that is—is replaced by the radically new P2. It does not seem that just any metaphysical accounts could map on to the theological claims, and some would seem to offer less cause for optimism (on Lockean accounts of personal identity, for instance, if psychological continuity is maintained then it is less than obvious that P2 would be distinct at all from P1—even if created out of nothing).[65] But perhaps—at least for the theologian who is

---

[63] Accordingly, we would read Paul's references to "the old person" (παλαιὸς ἡμῶν ἄνθρωπος) and "the body of sin" (σῶμα της ἁμαρτία) literally (Rom 6:6).

[64] On narrative self-constitution, see Marya Schectman, *The Constitution of Selves* (Ithaca: Cornell University Press, 1996), pp. 93–135. As she sees things, a "radical change in psychological organization involving the renunciation of a narrative sense of self, in effect, dismantles the person," but this does not amount to an endorsement of the claim (and related Buddhist views) on the question of "whether the personal self is, therefore, a fiction," p. 101. For perspective on the pre-philosophical appeal of narrative accounts, see John Bickle, "Empirical Evidence for a Narrative Concept of Self," in Gary D. Fireman, Ted E. McVay, Jr., Owen J. Flanagan, eds., *Narrative and Consciousness: Literature, Psychology, and the Brain* (Oxford: Oxford University Press, 2003), pp. 195–208. For criticisms of the narrative proposal, see Eric T. Olson and Karsten Witt, "Narrative and Persistence," *Canadian Journal of Philosophy* 49:3 (2019), pp. 419–434; John Christman, "Narrative Unity as a Condition of Personhood," *Metaphilosophy* 35:5 (2004), pp. 695–713; Lynne Rudder Baker, "Making Sense of Ourselves: Self-Narratives and Personal Identity," *Phenomenology and the Cognitive Sciences* 15:1 (2016), pp. 7–15.

[65] John Locke famously says that "personal identity consists, not in the Identity of Substance, but…in the Identity of *consciousness*," *An Essay Concerning Human Understanding*, P. Nidditch, ed. (Oxford: Oxford University Press, 1979), p. 342. Derek Parfit takes the criterion of personal identity over time to be:

willing to pay the metaphysical price—some local version of occasionalism offers a way forward.

Whatever we are to make of the RA view with respect to such matters, however, we are faced with some important theological concerns and challenges. The challenges come from several angles. At one level, the RA proposal is deeply counterintuitive. It is counterintuitive as a general account of reality. What Marya Schectman says about Derek Parfit's notion of teletransportation is relevant here too: this is "execution and replacement by a replica."[66] It is also counterintuitive as an interpretation of Galatians. Immediately, it seems clear that Paul is not reticent to talk about his own life from pre-conversion escapades to post-conversion union with Christ in terms of a stable and continuous personal identity. He recalls his own former way of life as someone who persecuted the ἐκκλησίαν τοῦ θεοῦ and tried to destroy it (1:13)—and he owns it *as his own*. From those days to his own stunning conversion to his meetings with Peter in Jerusalem and then to his own journeys as an evangelist and apostle of Jesus Christ, he recounts the story as one with undivided personal agency and apparent continuity of identity. Parfit says that "Identity is not what matters in survival."[67] But Paul would seem to think otherwise.

A concern stems from theological anthropology. For whatever we are to make of the more controverted elements of the passage, we must not lose sight of Paul's insistence on the importance of the *body*. As Paul puts it, the new life in Christ is life that is lived *in the flesh* (ἐν σαρκί). And it is a life that is lived *now* (νυν). In other words, the body—*this* flesh, *this* life lived in the body—matters to Paul. On the RA proposal, however, it would seem that the body fades in importance. For some versions of RA (including both physicalist and some dualist accounts), the body not only fades in importance but

---

The Psychological Criterion: (1) There is psychological continuity if and only if there are overlapping chains of strong connectedness. X today is one and the same person as Y at some past time if and only if (2) X is psychologically continuous with Y, (3) this continuity has the right kind of cause, and (4) there does not exist a different person who is psychologically continuous with Y. (5) Personal identity over time just consists in the holding of facts like (2) to (4).

Derek Parfit, *Reasons and Persons* (Oxford: Oxford University Press, 1984), p. 297.

[66]   Marya Schechtman, *The Constitution of Selves*, p. 22.

[67]   Parfit, *Reasons and Persons*, p. 217. Schectman notes that Parfit's claim is "deeply counterintuitive," *The Constitution of Selves*, p. 36. John Perry illustrates the counterintuitive nature vividly: "You learn that someone will be run over by a truck tomorrow; you are saddened, feel pity, and think reflectively about the frailty of life; one bit of information is added, that the someone is you, and a whole new set of emotions rise in your breast." John Perry, "The Importance of Being Identical," in A. Rorty, ed., *The Identities of Persons* (Berkeley: University of California Press, 1976), p. 67.

actually fades away entirely. The body that is the body of P1—for physical-
ists, the body that just *is* P1, and at any rate the body in which Paul (or any
person) lives as a sinner—is simply annihilated. It would seem that this body
is either not worth saving or, strictly speaking, is not salvageable.[68] This is a
remarkable un-Pauline conclusion, and thus should be unwelcome to
apocalyptic (as well as NPP and more traditional) interpreters.

A Christological concern is closely related. It plagues those apocalyptic
interpreters who also think that Christ assumed and has (or, during his
incarnate earthly career, *had*) a "fallen" or "sinful" human nature, and it is
especially intense for those who would also opt for a physicalist Christology.
Here is the problem in a nutshell, if Christ has a "fallen" human nature
(whatever exactly that means), and if the human body ($\sigma\alpha\rho\chi$) is destroyed
and replaced (as either not worth saving or not salvageable), then it would
seem that Christ's human body would also be left behind and replaced at his
resurrection and glorification. But if it is true that "the unassumed is the
unhealed," then the fact that Christ leaves behind his original human body
would be very bad news indeed. Moreover, on physicalist and occasionalist
assumptions, the Christ who is raised from the dead would not be the Christ
who died for us. For, again, while the Christ who suffered on the cross had a
fallen or sinful human nature, the new Christ would presumably be sinless,
and his humanity would be re-created *ex nihilo* after his old and sinful flesh
has been annihilated. On any plausible criteria of identity, it is not easy to see
how they might be identical. But Paul is absolutely convinced of the reality
of the bodily resurrection of Christ, and clearly he thinks that the person
who is the resurrected and exalted Christ is identical to the person who took
upon himself the form of a servant and became obedient to death on a cross
(1 Cor 15:12–28; Phil 2:5–11).

The RA proposal also raises some perplexing questions and worries
related to soteriology. Recall Linebaugh's anxiety over the criticisms of
Hampson. He asks if "soteriologies of death and resurrection – that is,
accounts of salvation like we encounter in Galatians and Luther's reading
of it – [are] finally opposed to the human person? Does the announcement
of the death of the I eliminate the possibility of God's love for the I? If I only

[68] On the other hand, if one were to adopt a more Cartesian version of the "local occasionalism" approach, the body might remain (even as the "person" or the "I" was replaced). But on
such a scenario it is again hard to see how the body really matters all that much, for the "real
person" (the immaterial soul) is completely replaced even though still stuck in the same body.
Again, on this view it would seem that the body is either not worth saving or not salvageable.

am outside myself and in Christ, does God ever look at and love me?"[69] Linebaugh's question is an important one. Linebaugh's own approach, as we have seen, merely asserts a "dialectical" conclusion: there both is and is not an "I" that is loved and saved by God. As we have also seen, this approach is unsatisfactory, for to assert that in the same sense there both *is* and *is not* an "I" that is continuously loved and finally saved is only to assert a contradiction. Since contradictions are necessarily false, this is not a good option. The question itself remains, however, and it is troubling. So, is there—or is there not—an I that is always loved and finally saved? If the answer is No, then there is no hope of salvation. If the answer is Yes, on the other hand, then it is hard to see how the RA proposal can be right.

Further questions arise. Am "I" joined in union with Christ—or am "I" not? Earlier the concern had to do with the identity of the incarnate Christ, but here we have a similar worry about the identity of the person who is said to be joined to Christ. Paul claims to be crucified *with* Christ. Is the Paul who has new life the one who was co-crucified with Christ? The verb used (συνεσταύρωμαι) is in the perfect tense. Some commentators take this to indicate that Paul's statement refers to a once-for-all act of committed faith that joins the believer in union with Christ with "results and implications for the present."[70] Other scholars take the force of the perfect tense to signal something rather stronger; thus Andrew Das takes it to refer to an "on-going state of co-crucifixion with Christ," and James D. G. Dunn says that the one who is co-crucified continues "in that state, still hanging on the cross."[71] Dunn explains his view: "Paul did not think of crucifixion with Christ as a once-for-all event of the past. Nor was he thinking in these passages of the believer as already taken down from the cross and risen with Christ. On the contrary . . . I have been nailed to the cross with Christ, and am in that state still; *I am hanging with Christ on that cross.* The implication for the process of salvation is clear: since the resurrection with Christ comes at the end point, then in a sense (in terms of soteriological effect) Christ remains the crucified one until the parousia, and those crucified with Christ continue to

[69] Linebaugh, "The Speech of the Dead," p. 103.

[70] E.g., Richard N. Longenecker, *Galatians*, Word Biblical Commentary 41 (Grand Rapids: Zondervan Academic,1990), p. 92; Tarzi, *Galatians*, p. 88; Ben Witherington III, *Grace in Galatia: A Commentary on Paul's Letter to the Galatians* (Edinburgh: T&T Clark, 1998), p. 190.

[71] A. Andrew Das, *Galatians* (St. Louis: Concordia Publishing House, 2014), p. 268; James D. G. Dunn, *The Theology of Paul's Letter to the Galatians* (Cambridge: Cambridge University Press, 1993), p. 120.

be crucified with Christ throughout the period of overlap."[72] But either way we take it, either as a once-for-all event with continuing impact or as a continuing activity, the claim does not sit well with the RA proposal. For if we take it in the stronger sense suggested by Dunn, the process described is continuous and ongoing. Thus there must be direct and straightforward continuity of the person throughout the entire process and indeed all the way until the parousia. Suppose, on the other hand, that we opt for the view that this expresses a once-for-all event. On this reading too, however, what happens in this once-for-all event has ongoing significance for the present precisely because it is the same person or "I." So either way, the RA proposal faces an exegetical challenge.

It is worth noting that such exegetical and doctrinal concerns are accompanied by some pressing pastoral and existential worries. Campbell says that the fact that Jesus Christ "had to die, executing our *condition*, then resurrecting human nature *in a new form*, suggests that there was something irredeemably corrupt and contaminated in the old one," and he concludes that "our problem goes down into the very roots of our nature."[73] With this claim in mind, let us return to the concerns expressed by Hampson. Hampson is opposed to notions of co-crucifixion and, more broadly, surrender and death; on behalf of people who have been oppressed and abused, she protests that such persons are further damaged by any theology that tells them that what they need is to be broken and replaced. She is convinced that such doctrine only brings further damage to those marginalized and oppressed persons who have been robbed of any proper sense of self.[74] Such concerns are important for more traditional theologians and the proponents of the NPP too, and they deserve a hearing. But it is not easy to see how the RA proposal has much in the way of resources for responding to them. After all, if the *I*—the *self* or the *person*—is annihilated, then surely she loses her identity. She might not want to hear that she *needs* to be saved in any case, but it is not hard to understand how she might conclude that this "gospel" tells her that she is "irredeemably corrupt and contaminated," either not worth saving or not salvageable.

---

[72] James D. G. Dunn, *Theology of Paul the Apostle* (Grand Rapids: William B. Eerdmans Publishing Co., 1998), p. 485.

[73] Douglas Campbell, *Pauline Dogmatics* (Grand Rapids: William B. Eerdmans Publishing Co., 2020), p. 116 n7.

[74] See Daphne Hampson, *Christian Contradictions: The Structures of Lutheran and Catholic Thought* (Cambridge: Cambridge University Press, 2001), pp. 237–241, and Daphne Hampson, "Luther on the Self: A Feminist Critique," *Word and World* 8:4 (1988), pp. 334–342.

1.3.2 Fusion Theories

There might be another option for apocalyptic theologians who insist on such radical discontinuity between the old and the new. Some statements from various apocalyptic interpreters might be taken to suggest something rather different and perhaps even more radical yet; instead of an annihilation and replacement, we might have something more like absorption or fusion with Christ. Recall Barclay's claim that those who are baptized "into Christ" now "constitute one person." And consider further Das's claim that Paul is not talking about an "'I' [that] operates alongside the agency of Christ, 'but that Christ operates in and even as the human agent."[75] Taken with meta-physical seriousness, this might be taken to suggest a kind of fusion.[76] On such a proposal, perhaps there are many persons who exist as individuals before the co-crucifixion event, but at this event they lose distinct identity and instead become one person. Indeed, they become the one person who is Christ. Accordingly, after the co-crucifixion event the person of Christ is now the *only* person,[77] for the person of Christ is now a sort of super-person who has temporal parts that once were personally distinct.[78]

1.3.2.1 The Theory of Final Assumptions

One option—probably the best option—for fusionists is the "theory of final assumptions" (TFA) that has been offered by Thomas P. Flint.[79] Galatians 2:20 is not offered as any sort of "proof-text" of the theory (although Flint does mention it as possible support), and Flint offers TFA only as specula-tion.[80] The theory is summarized neatly by Flint: "The ultimate end of all human beings who attain salvation is to be assumed by the Son."[81] Flint is

---

[75] Das, *Galatians*, p. 270.

[76] See the discussion of fusion and personal identity in Derek Parfit, "Personal Identity," *Philosophical Review* 80:1 (1971), pp. 18–21.

[77] At least for those proponents of RA who are also universalists with respect to salvation. Alternatively, all of the redeemed come to constitute one person by fusion with Jesus Christ.

[78] Such an approach would have a nice symmetry with "fission" versions of realist doctrines of original sin, on which see Michael C. Rea, "The Metaphysics of Original Sin," in Peter van Inwagen and Dean Zimmerman, eds., *Persons, Divine and Human* (Oxford: Oxford University Press, 2007), pp. 341–345; and Hud Hudson, "Fission, Freedom, and the Fall," in Jonathan L. Kvanvig ed., *Oxford Studies in Philosophy of Religion* Vol. 2 (Oxford: Oxford University Press, 2009), pp. 58–79.

[79] Thanks to Oliver D. Crisp for suggesting this as a possibility.

[80] Thomas P. Flint, "Molinism and Incarnation," in Ken Perszyk, ed., *Molinism: The Contemporary Debate* (Oxford: Oxford University Press, 2011), p. 199.

[81] Flint, "Molinism and Incarnation," p. 198.

clear about what he means by "assumption," he intends to affirm nothing less than that God actually becomes incarnate in each human person who is redeemed by God. As he explains, TFA is the view that

> for the elect, this union will ultimately become as metaphysically real as is the union between CHN [Christ's human nature, commonly understood as the body-soul composite of the incarnate Son] and the Son. During our lives on earth, most of us make fitful and imperfect progress toward this union. But the grace of God is stronger than our weakness, and can eventually (if we do not resist its influence) re-make us more completely in this image and likeness of God. When this process has reached the appropriate stage, after many struggles here on earth (and perhaps further purgation after death), God sees that we have been made worthy of our final goal. At that point, the Son assumes us, and we become united to him as truly and completely as CHN has always been united to him. God becomes incarnate in each of us.[82]

Flint notes that this assumption happens "at the appropriate stage," and, as he explains it, this stage is reached when the "process of sanctification" reaches a point at which the redeemed person no longer sins and will not sin again.[83]

1.3.2.2 Too Many Persons?

While intriguing, the TFA is not without challenges. Here are three: the "too many persons" worry, the "too many natures" worry, and the "too many sinners" worry. The "too many persons" worry is concerned that the TFA leaves us with too many incarnate persons. The TFA can, of course, deny that there is more than one incarnate person. And the TFA *should* do so, at least if it wants to maintain consistency with conciliar Christology.[84] After all, Chalcedon decrees that there is "one Person" in the incarnation.[85] However, the theory does not claim that there are multiple incarnate human persons, but that the one incarnate person assumes multiple human natures (where those are understood "concretely"; again, for much of the tradition, as a unique body-soul composite). So, in addition to CHN,

---

[82] Flint, "Molinism and Incarnation," p. 198.
[83] Flint, "Molinism and Incarnation," p. 198.
[84] On "conciliar Christology," see Timothy Pawl, *In Defense of Conciliar Christology: A Philosophical Essay* (Oxford: Oxford University Press, 2016), especially pp. 11–28.
[85] "The Chalcedonian Decree," in Edward Rochie Hardy, ed., *The Christology of the Later Fathers* (Louisville: Westminster John Knox Press, 1977), p. 373.

the Son assumes Paul's human nature (PHN).[86] Incarnate only as Jesus Christ, what we have is CHN+Son; this is one person. Once Paul is assumed, what we have is Son+CHN+PHN, but still as one person.

Or do we? With the assumption of PHN, do we still have *Paul*, or do we not? If Paul is no longer in the picture, we are left to wonder just who it is that continues to refer to himself as Paul (cf. Phil 1:1; and assuming the standard critical view that Philippians postdates Galatians). If it is not Paul, then is it PHN? How can PHN do the talking if already de-personalized? At this point, we do not know enough. If Paul is in the picture, then just what is Paul? If Paul is a person—while making the claims of Gal 2:20 and thus, on this theory, incarnate—then we have too many persons. On the other hand, if the co-crucified "I" is really the person who is Son+CHN+PHN, then the only *person* here is the Son. But then who is talking to whom when Paul prays to Jesus (e.g., 1 Cor 1:2; 16:22)? If the co-crucified "Paul" is a de-personalized PHN who nonetheless acts as an agent and prays to Jesus and talks about being co-crucified, then it is hard to distinguish PHN from plain old Paul. "They" look like the self-same person.[87] To make progress here, it seems that we need a supporting story to tell of how Paul is de-personalized (perhaps a sort of *exhypostasis* to accompany the traditional distinction between *anhypostasis* and *enhypostasis*). For without that, it is really hard to distinguish Paul as a person acting as a speech-agent from PHN acting as a speech-agent.

Peter van Inwagen holds that persons "are those things to which personal pronouns are applicable: a person can use the word 'I' and be addressed as a 'thou.'"[88] For those whose intuitions align with van Inwagen on this point, any alleged distinctions between some PHN who can use personal indexicals and Paul himself will likely look like a distinction without a difference. Moreover, as Flint himself observes, TFA entails that persons are not essentially persons. Flint also notes it is very counterintuitive (some might say *wildly* so) to think that a person is not a person essentially. Alfred

[86] And—hopefully, on this theory—many, many others as well.

[87] While more pronounced, the concern here is similar to the one that attaches to the proposal that "person-stages" can be distinguished from persons. As David Lewis says of "person-stages": a person-stage does "many of the same things that a person does; it talks and walks and thinks, it has beliefs and desires, it has a size and shape and location..." David Lewis, "Survival and Identity," in *Philosophical Papers*, vol. 1 (Oxford: Oxford University Press, 1983). Harold Noonan notes that it "might be hard to deny that person-stages *are* persons," for they "walk and talk and think, and have beliefs and desires" and leave us asking "What more could one ask?" for personhood. Harold Noonan, *Personal Identity* (London: Routledge, 1991), p. 126.

[88] See the discussion in Peter van Inwagen, *God, Knowledge, and Mystery: Essays in Philosophical Theology* (Ithaca: Cornell University Press, 1995), pp. 265–267.

J. Freddoso says that he finds this "extraordinarily implausible"; it is a "manifest repugnancy which flouts our deepest convictions about ourselves" and is "utterly bereft of merit."[89] Flint disagrees, of course, and the debates over this issue would take us far afield. But those who are on Team Freddoso on this point will see this as a serious problem with the proposal.

Now perhaps the proponents of RA will not be dislodged by such objections based on appeals to intuitions (even intuitions about identity and modality that are both very common and very powerful). Perhaps some proponents of RA will even take extraordinary implausibility as a badge of honor. After all, if it is true, as Barclay claims, that "the cross of Christ shatters every ordered system of norms, however embedded in the 'natural' order of 'the world,'" then we should not be at all surprised or dismayed by the fact that the apocalyptic gospel of Christ "flouts our deepest convictions about ourselves."[90] Perhaps it is a good thing to be "utterly bereft of merit," for, according to apocalypticism, both revelation and salvation are completely by grace.

To be clear, I have presented the "too many persons" worry as just that—a worry. I do not serve this up as a fatal objection or as a charge of heresy. But it is a worry that should, I think, really concern the proponents of RA who might be attracted to the TFA. For those who think of persons as van Inwagen does, it is not easy to know the difference between the person who is Paul and the non-person who is PHN but looks and sounds and acts just like Paul. For those who think of persons as the kind of things that are essentially persons (as does Freddoso), then the alignment of TFA with RA will be a complete non-starter. And, more broadly, the TFA does not seem to align well with what Paul is saying here. When Paul refers to the "life I now live in the flesh" (ὃ δὲ νῦν ζῶ ἐν σαρκί), the verb he uses is a present active indicative. Again, just who is this? It can't be the person who is Paul, for then we would have two incarnate persons and thus would violate conciliar Christology. So is it the person who is the Son (+CHN+PHN)? But then who is he talking to? Or is it PHN—but then how is this any different than the person who is Paul? Minimally, we need more explanation.

1.3.2.3 Too Many Natures?
Famously, conciliar Christology holds to the "double *homoousion*"; the incarnate Son is both consubstantial with the Father and consubstantial

[89] Alfred J. Freddoso, "Human Nature, Potency, and the Incarnation," *Faith and Philosophy* 3:1 (1986), p. 37.

[90] Barclay, *Paul and the Gift*, p. 394.

with humans. This means that the Son is to be "acknowledged in two natures."[91] Some of the familiar challenges to classical Christology (e.g., adoptionism, Eutychianism) threatened this affirmation by reducing the number of natures to one. On the TFA, however, it appears that we have a different problem. It looks like we have more than two natures. Indeed, it turns out that the incarnate Son has *many* natures. With respect to this passage (interpreted along the lines of RA bolstered by a fusionist TFA), there are three natures on display: the divine nature of the Son, CHN, and PHN. On the face of it, at least, this is one nature too many.

A defender of the RA-TFA view might respond by saying that what the venerable ecumenical statement means is "*at least* two natures," so that a position that holds to "two-or-more" natures might be acceptable. But of course this is not what the official statement says, and I know of no major patristic or medieval interpreter of the creed who took it this way. Recall the parallel affirmation that the incarnate Son is *one person*. Surely no one would take seriously a retort (perhaps from Nestorians) that goes along the lines of "well, the creed never says '*exactly one person*.' So it must just mean '*at least one person*,' and any position that holds to 'one-or-more-persons' is acceptable by the standards of the creeds." By parity, neither should we adopt a "two-or-more" natures reading of the creed. At best such a reading is implausible. Alternatively, one might say that what the creed demands is only the confession that the incarnate Son has an *abstract* (rather than concrete) human nature. If so, then, by being incarnate, the Son has exactly two abstract natures—one divine and one human—and he has the abstract human nature by exemplifying multiple concrete human natures. Accordingly, the desideratum of the creed is satisfied so long as Christ has at least one concrete human nature, and it does not really matter (for purposes of satisfying the creed) how many of those he has. This may be a way forward (the debates between concretists and abstractists are longstanding, of course), but it seems to me that anyone who takes this view of the creedal statements loses significant support for concretism. At any rate, again, more explanation would be helpful.

1.3.2.4 Too Many Sinners?
So far, we have faced concerns about both the possibility that the TFA leaves us with too many natures, and further that thinking of those natures as

[91] "The Chalcedonian Decree," p. 373.

agents seems to leave us with too many persons. There is a further worry, and the concern here is about just what those agents (whether understood as persons or de-personed natures) are *doing* with their agency. This is the "too many sinners" worry. Flint is aware of this concern; as he expresses it: "If we let X stand for some human nature, it will be true to say in heaven that X sinned. And if X has been assumed by the Son, it follows that it will also be true to say that the Son sinned."[92] He thinks that this is an "intriguing objection," but he thinks that it can be handled the way that one handles other seemingly incompatible Christological predicates. As the Son is limited in knowledge (according to CHN) but omniscient (according to the divine nature), so also the Son can be said to be have the property of necessary goodness (and thus impeccability) according to the divine nature but also the property of *having sinned* (according to PHN). Thus, on TFA it is "true to say that the Son sinned, but only in a borrowed sense."[93] Flint thinks that this is enough to avoid any heterodox or otherwise untoward consequences.

Flint may or may not be correct about this worry when applied to the TFA in a stand-alone sense.[94] It may be that the "too many sinners" worry threatens not a stand-alone TFA proposal but only the alliance of TFA with RA as a reading of Galatians 2:20 (as Flint seems to suggest).[95] The reason that it may threaten an alliance of TFA but perhaps not TFA itself has to do with timing; Flint's TFA seems to assume an eschatological terminus for redeemed humans as incarnate, but Paul's statement is about what is happening "*now*." The challenge should be obvious: if anyone who is joined in union with Christ is the same person as Christ and then commits sin, then the person who is the divine Son sins. This is hardly a property that is "borrowed" in the sense that it attaches to something that happened earlier in the life of a formerly hypostasized nature (or a property that attaches to the whole in virtue of being a property of an earlier temporal part that was assumed at a later time); this is something that happens *now* and is currently the action of the person. Whatever we are to make of Flint's metaphysics, the conclusion with which we are left appears to contradict creedal and biblical statements. For Chalcedon says that the incarnate Son is "like us in all things

---

[92] Flint, "Molinism and Incarnation," p. 201.
[93] Flint, "Molinism and Incarnation," p. 202.
[94] For reasons that would take us afield, I am not convinced that his proposed strategy does enough.
[95] More precisely, Flint suggests that this passage might provide support for TFA, but he does not mention apocalyptic theology.

except sin."[96] And Chalcedon is only echoing Hebrews 4:15 at this point: "For we do not have a high priest who is unable to sympathize with our weaknesses, but we have one who in every respect has been tested as we are, yet without sin."

At any rate, it is not obvious that TFA will be attractive to the proponents of the RA position. For Barclay himself also says that Paul has "no hesitation in speaking of the believers as agents."[97] Das adds that nothing in the process is "obliterating their capacity to act."[98] Campbell says that Paul "is still distinguishable as a person within this progress."[99] So while it is a fascinating proposal and may offer the best way forward for RA, nonetheless it is beset with challenges.

1.4 A Traditional Interpretation Reconsidered

It is not uncommon for apocalyptic interpreters to be critical or even dismissive of traditional interpretations. Linebaugh, as we have seen, rejects Aquinas's account as a misguided effort to "domesticate" the true gospel. The basic interpretation offered by Aquinas, however, is not at all unique to him. To the contrary, it shares much in common with views that are much older.

Moving from such generalities to more focused exegetical considerations, let us consider John Chrysostom's interpretation of the passage. Chrysostom seems to take Paul's claim to have "died to the Law" through or by means of the Law to be nothing short of autobiographical. He also finds the claim rather ambiguous, and he lays out three possible interpretations. First, dying *to* the Law by means of the Law might refer in the first use of the term to the Mosaic law and in the second use to the "law of grace," to what Paul refers to elsewhere as "the law of the Spirit of life" (Rom 8:2). The second option is this: dying to the Law by means of the Law might refer to the fact that the Mosaic law itself points beyond itself and indicates that we should obey Christ rather than the law. A third option is to understand this as the recognition that the law places all those who do not fulfill it completely under sentence of death while also showing us that no one fulfills it completely (cf. Rom 3:23). Chrysostom explores these options but then seems to incline toward the third. He notes that Paul does *not* say "the Law is dead to me"; instead he says "I am dead to the Law," and he takes

---

[96] "The Chalcedonian Decree," p. 373.   [97] Barclay, *Paul and the Gift*, p. 441.
[98] Das, *Galatians*, p. 270.   [99] Campbell, *The Justification of God*, p. 848.

the meaning of this to be that "as it is impossible for a dead corpse to obey the commands of the Law, so also is it for me who have perished by its curse, for by its word I am slain."[100]

Chrysostom takes the death to refer primarily to spiritual death (although with what he takes to be obvious implications for physical life and death), and he takes the new life now "lived unto God" to be immortal and thus spiritual life (although, again, with what he takes to be obvious implications for physical life and death). Paul's claim to be co-crucified is understood by Chrysostom to refer to union with Christ in baptism, and the words "nevertheless I live, yet not I" refer to "our subsequent manner of life whereby our members are mortified."[101] When Paul says that Christ lives in him, he means that he does nothing of which Christ would disapprove. For as Paul's reference to "death" here "signifies not what is commonly understood" but a "death to sin," so also by "life" he means "a delivery from sin."[102] Chrysostom explains that someone "cannot live to God, otherwise than by dying to sin, and as Christ suffered bodily death, so does Paul [undergo] a death to sin."[103] Chrysostom takes this to be an event that is in some sense past and settled, for at baptism the "old man" ($\pi\alpha\lambda\alpha\iota\grave{o}s$ $\mathring{\eta}\mu\hat{\omega}\nu$ $\mathring{\alpha}\nu\theta\rho\omega\pi\sigma s$) was crucified (Rom 6:6).[104] But he also takes it to be something that continues to involve our active commitment and participation. Thus Paul calls upon believers to put to death fornication, uncleanness, and passion (Col 3:5); one remains alive to God so long as one is dead to sin, but to allow sin to live again is to bring ruin to the new life.[105] Chrysostom calls upon his readers to recognize the perfection of Paul's walk with Christ, for Paul's "universal obedience" to God's will enables him to say "not, 'I live to Christ' but, 'Christ lives in me.'"[106]

How does this interpretation compare to the RA proposal? Before proceeding, we should be clear about how mainstream traditional interpretations (such as Chrysostom's) are in agreement with apocalyptic accounts. As Paul D. Murray points out, for many theological interpreters of Paul in the tradition (he focuses upon Augustine and Aquinas), "the entirety of

[100] John Chrysostom, "Commentary on Galatians," in Philip Schaff, ed., *A Select Library of the Nicene and Post-Nicene Fathers of the Christian Church* Vol. XIII (Grand Rapids: William B. Eerdmans Publishing Co., 1994), p. 22.
[101] Chrysostom, "Commentary on Galatians," p. 22.
[102] Chrysostom, "Commentary on Galatians," p. 22.
[103] Chrysostom, "Commentary on Galatians," p. 22.
[104] Chrysostom, "Commentary on Galatians," p. 22.
[105] Chrysostom, "Commentary on Galatians," p. 22.
[106] Chrysostom, "Commentary on Galatians," p. 22.

Christian life, from beginning to end and all between, is throughout and at once grace-initiated, grace-situated and grace-drawn; grace-held and grace-impelled…"[107] So, for traditional as well as apocalyptic interpreters, the primacy and necessity of grace is not in question. We can, however, see differences in several respects. First, and fundamentally, the older reading maintains straightforward ontological continuity between the "I" who lived before and then was crucified with Christ and the "I" who now lives in union with Christ. Where the RA proposal posits a sharp and definitive break between the old and the new, Chrysostom never doubts that there is a robust continuity. Thus, he feels no need to struggle with the qualms that bother Linebaugh; he simply knows that God loved *him*, that Christ died for *him*, and that *his* new life is found in union with Christ. Second, Chrysostom's interpretation understands this "I"—the one that retains identity from old to new—to be decisively transformed. He takes the "death" referred to by Paul to be the cessation of the former way of life and the new life to be a life that is now "dead to sin" and instead vivified by God. He notes that Paul's claim is not "I live to Christ"; it is not as if this is an effort at self-renovation. It is not something that can be reduced to moralism. Instead, Chrysostom points out, Paul's astounding claim is that "Christ lives in me."[108] Third, Chrysostom also understands this new life to be just that—an ongoing, full-orbed, robust *life*. He is not thinking of some sort of static or legal condition. The older views are sometimes criticized by their apocalyptic critics for narrowing down salvation to a legal declaration. Meanwhile, as we have seen, the RA view raises questions about the place of human agency and the transform-ation of human agents. Chrysostom's view is different; his is an optimism of grace, and it is deeply theological and Christological in its basis and trans-formational in nature. For he sees crucifixion with Christ as something that involves and transforms the entire person; affections are transformed and actions are changed. Finally, his view takes the work of God in Christ and the new life provided by it to be both universal and particular as well as unconditional in one sense but conditional in another. Some versions of the older (especially "Reformed") views are the focus of criticism for limiting the extent of God's work in Christ, and, conversely, some expressions of the RA proposal raise concerns about the place and importance of human response.

[107] Paul D. Murray, "Thomas Aquinas and the Potential Catholic Integration of a Dynamic Occasionalist Understanding of Grace," *International Journal of Systematic Theology* 22:1 (2020), p. 91.
[108] Chrysostom, "Commentary on Galatians," p. 22.

Chrysostom's interpretation differs from both in important ways. He clearly thinks of God's work in Christ to be, in important senses, both universal and unconditional. What Christ does is intended for, and available to, all. At the same time, however, in another sense what God does in the event of Christ's crucifixion is both particular and conditional, for it both invites and requires a response. As the "Golden-Mouthed" preacher puts it, "the sacrifice was offered for all . . . and sufficient to save all, but those who enjoy the blessing are the believing only."[109]

1.5 Crucified with Christ: A Modest Proposal

What are we to make of all this? I began with a comparison of what I have called the "Modest" and "Radical" apocalyptic interpretations of Paul. I confess that I am convinced by the Radical proposal that the "nomistic" interpretation offered by the Modesty crowd does not do justice to the point that Paul makes with such force and passion. I think that we are indebted to the Radical proponents for insisting that Paul's account demands more than this. But I have also argued that the Radical reading runs into serious difficulties. The debates over these matters are likely to continue, but I think that the difficulties I have spelled out make it untenable. On the other hand, I find that the older interpretation represented by John Chrysostom avoids such problems while also steering clear of the merely "nomistic self" interpretation. Briefly, I shall summarize the main points.

First, it seems obvious that there is ontological continuity of the self; however exactly we are to account for this metaphysically, there is real personal identity of the pre-conversion Paul and the post-conversion Paul.[110] We might follow Kathryn Tanner in saying that "the grace that changes us has its *analogue* in the divine acts that created us – from nothing" and that this transformation is "*like* the rebirth from the dead."[111] But in

---

[109] Chrysostom, "Commentary on Galatians," p. 23.

[110] For present purposes, we need not endorse any particular view; whether one opts for, say, four-dimensionalism over other proposals will depend upon other factors. As Marya Schectman summarizes matters, four-dimensionalists are those who "believe that a person is *never wholly present* at any one time, but only over time, and that person-stages are parts out of which continuant persons are composed." Three-dimensionalists, on the other hand, "believe persons are three-dimensional enduring objects" who are "wholly present at each time in [their] history, and time-slices of that history are not to be viewed as genuine *parts* of a person." Marya Schectman, *The Constitution of Selves*, p. 11.

[111] Kathryn Tanner, *Christ the Key* (Cambridge: Cambridge University Press, 2010), pp. 64–65, emphasis mine.

doing so, it is important to maintain real personal identity. For as Susan G. Eastman puts it, "the power of God works in his life without obliterating his 'self' (2:20)." To the contrary, as she rightly notes, "the power of God frees Paul to be an agent, an acting subject" in ways that he was unable to before.[112]

Second, the death referred to here is not total annihilation. It is not a cessation of being or the loss or replacement of personal identity. Instead, to "die" here refers to the surrender of the former and sinful way of life.[113] As Wright says, "dying to something" means "repudiating it."[114]

Third, the new life that is lived in union with Christ is life that is morally transformed. As Michael J. Gorman observes, Paul places great importance on the reality of life that is transformed in light of the resurrection.[115] There are, as Walter Hansen points out, both passive and active elements to Paul's teaching.[116] The ethical elements are holistic in nature; Paul insists that this is life that is lived now ($\nu\nu\nu$). And it is life that is lived in the "flesh" ($\sigma\alpha\rho\chi$). "Flesh" here does not carry the negative connotations that it does elsewhere in Paul. In fact, it is striking that Paul opts for this word to describe the new life that is lived "*now*." His view of the power of the crucified and resurrected Son of God is so strong that he believes that even our "flesh" is redeemed and restored and eventually perfected. In Paul's usage here, "flesh" is, as de Boer puts it, merely "the substance that covers a human being's bones."[117] As such, this fleshly, embodied existence may still be mortal and weak, but it is not sinful as such. As Eastman says, Paul is referring "simply to human, corporeal existence."[118] The importance of this is profound: Paul is not saying that deliverance from evil comes only at the last day or at some point when those redeemed by God will have different bodies or completely new identities. No, he is saying that the life that is lived now—the life lived in *this* flesh—is life that is lived in union with Christ.

As such, this life that is lived in union with Christ shares the "mind of Christ." Recent work on "joint attention" is relevant here.[119] What Paul

[112] Susan G. Eastman, *Recovering Paul's Mother Tongue: Language and Theology in Galatians* (Grand Rapids: William B. Eerdmans Publishing Co., 2007), p. 60.

[113] Richard Longenecker, *Galatians*, p. 91.

[114] N. T. Wright, *Paul and the Faithfulness of God* (Minneapolis: Fortress Press, 2013), p. 1430.

[115] Michael J. Gorman, *Inhabiting the Cruciform God: Kenosis, Justification, and Theosis in Paul's Narrative Soteriology* (Grand Rapids: William B. Eerdmans Publishing Co., 2009), p. 67.

[116] Walter Hansen, *Galatians* (Downers Grove: InterVarsity Academic, 2010), p. 76.

[117] de Boer, *Galatians*, p. 162.   [118] Eastman, *Paul's Mother Tongue*, p. 168.

[119] Similarly, something akin to Schectman's account "empathic access" is important here, but I say "something akin" because while her proposal is oriented toward "affective connection

gestures toward here is not merely a collection of third-person statements *about* Christ, but nor, as Eastman points out, does Paul mean to indicate that his union with Christ is "an extension of first-person self-awareness."[120] It is, instead, something more like "joint attention." As such, it includes both what Eleonore Stump refers to as "dyadic joint attention" and what she calls "triadic joint attention."[121] Dyadic joint attention refers to the mutual closeness and shared presence of two persons in relation to one another; in our case, it would refer to the shared attention whereby Paul and Christ know one another to such an extent that Paul and Christ come to share the same affections and intentions. Thus Paul comes to know—even if imperfectly, yet more and more—what Christ values, what Christ loathes, and what Christ loves. Paul's knowledge of this is *personal* knowledge, and Paul comes to know this about Christ only as he comes to *share* the affections and intentions of Christ. For Paul to be joined in union with Christ is for Paul to know and share Christ's own passion for justice and mercy. It is to know and share the "wrath of the Lamb" against all that despoils God's good creation and especially those creatures made in God's image. It is to know and share Christ's love for those who have been bruised and busted and broken by sin.

Such joint attention that comes with union with Christ also involves a triadic dimension. This is shared focus and mutual intentions toward a third party or person; in our case, it would refer to the shared attention that Paul and Christ direct toward *another*. Thus Paul comes to know—even if imperfectly, yet more and more—Christ's devotion to God and his intentions for the creation. Again, Paul's knowledge of this is *personal* knowledge, and Paul comes to know this as he comes to actually *share* Christ's affections and intentions. With Christ, Paul comes to know and share the communion of the Son with the Father in the fellowship of the Holy Spirit. With Christ, Paul comes to know and share Christ's compassion for his creatures and indeed in his willingness to suffer for the sake of his enemies. As Paul

---

to the past, together with its behavioral implications," the Christian account of new life in union with Christ would include a strong "affective connection" both to *Christ's past* and one's own future existence lived in union with Christ. See Marya Schectman, "Empathic Access: The Missing Ingredient in Personal Identity," *Philosophical Explorations* 4:2 (2001), p. 102.

[120] Susan Grove Eastman, "Knowing and Being Known: Interpersonal Cognition and the Knowledge of God," in Andrew B. Torrance and Thomas H. McCall, eds., *Knowing Creation: Perspectives from Theology, Philosophy, and Science* (Grand Rapids: Zondervan Academic, 2018), p. 157.

[121] Eleonore Stump, *Wandering in Darkness: Narrative and the Problem of Suffering* (Oxford: Oxford University Press, 2010), pp. 113–119. See also Eleonore Stump, "Omnipresence, Indwelling, and the Second-Personal," *European Journal for Philosophy of Religion* (2013), pp. 29–53; Susan G. Eastman, "The Shadow Side of Second-Person Engagement: Sin in Paul's Letter to the Romans," *European Journal for Philosophy of Religion* (2013), pp. 125–144.

comes to know Christ's love more and more, so also he comes to share Christ's desire not only for the good of the other but also a desire for union with the other.

The proposal I am offering here coheres well with the deep-seated and widespread intuition that morality is central to notions of self-understanding and our sense of our selves. As Nina Strohminger and Shaun Nichols have argued, very common intuitions pump out the conclusion that "moral traits are considered more important to personal identity than any other part of the mind."[122] Indeed, these intuitions are so strong that it is natural to refer to someone who has been renovated and remade morally and spiritually as a "new person." This is no less powerful for being non-literal. On the proposal that I am forwarding, the same person or self or "I" has been renewed so thoroughly and sanctified so wholly that she rightly can be said to be a "new creature" in a crucially important sense (2 Cor 5:17)—but while maintaining ontological continuity rather than being de-personalized or demolished and then replaced.

What I am proposing also intersects with insights that are available from "narrative" accounts of identity.[123] On narrative accounts, personal identity is shaped by the stories that one inhabits and the communities that tell those stories. As Hilde Lindemann Nelson puts it, personal identity "embodies an understanding" that is shaped and sculpted by "one's own and others's selective, interpretive, and connective representations of the characteristics, acts, experiences, roles, relationships, and commitments that contribute importantly to one's life over time, an identity that makes a certain sort of sense of who one is," and thus one's personal identity is "essentially narrative in nature."[124] "Master narratives" are those that are put upon us; they are the stories in which we find ourselves and often accept as definitive for our understandings of our roles and indeed of our very selves. They are also, sadly, often oppressive, and they can be instruments of enslavement. Identities, says Nelson, are "damaged when powerful institutions or individuals, seeing people as...moral sub- or abnormal, unjustly prevent" a person from roles and relationships wherein they would flourish.[125] This

---

[122] Nina Strohminger and Shaun Nichols, "The Essential Moral Self," *Cognition* 131:1 (2014), p. 168. I should note that "widespread" and "very common" is indexed to empirical work among North Americans in the early twenty-first century.

[123] I do not endorse such narrative accounts as full or complete accounts of personal identity.

[124] Hilde Lindemann Nelson, *Damaged Identities, Narrative Repair* (Ithaca: Cornell University Press, 2001), p. 15.

[125] Nelson, *Damaged Identities*, p. 20.

occurs through "deprivation of opportunity," but it goes much deeper when the damaged and oppressed person accepts the account of the master narrative and comes to have an "infiltrated consciousness."[126]

"Counterstories," on the other hand, "are stories of self-definition."[127] As such, they serve to define one's own present identity, but they also have the capacity to define not only the past and even to shape the future.[128] As such, they hold the potential for "narrative repair" whereby a person comes to accept and live into the roles and relationships wherein she will flourish. Significantly, such "counterstories can be created *by* or *for* the person whose identity needs repair."[129]

Understood in a narrative register, Paul's confession can be seen initially to follow a master narrative. It is one in which he is not said to be the oppressed but indeed is said to be the *oppressor* (Gal 1:13–14). He is brought into a counterstory when God "revealed" the Son (Gal 1:11–12, 15–16). This counterstory is not one of his own making but is radically unexpected and unsettling. It is one that is definitively "created *for* the person whose identity needs repair." It makes Paul what he ought to be, and as Paul comes to share joint attention with Christ and thus has the "mind of Christ," he finally flourishes. But Paul's account is different too—the story of Christ into which Paul is joined (when he is joined in union with the person that is Christ) is the counterstory that brings "repair" to Paul as Paul is *both* crucified with and risen with Christ. And where Nelson's account of narrative repair "allows oppressed people to refuse the identities imposed on them by their oppressors and to reidentify themselves in more respectworthy terms," Paul's own story is radically different.[130] For Paul is not merely transformed from *oppressed victim* to flourishing person, he is transformed from *haughty oppressor* to one whose own life is now one of love and gift (Gal 2:20). For "where sin increased, grace abounded all the more" (Rom 5:20).

Despite these strengths, however, does such a proposal—one that looks backward to go forward—somehow "domesticate" the gospel? Does my admittedly traditional reading somehow undercut the "singularity" and "radicality" of the one true gospel proclaimed by Paul? I cannot see how it does. To the contrary, I am awestruck by the power and radicality of it. I take it that what Paul is talking about here is his account of his own personal experience, but it is more than that. It is, as Wright points out, a "paradigm

---

[126] Nelson, *Damaged Identities*, p. 21.   [127] Nelson, *Damaged Identities*, p. 15.
[128] Nelson, *Damaged Identities*, pp. 17–18.   [129] Nelson, *Damaged Identities*, p. 19.
[130] Nelson, *Damaged Identities*, p. 22.

case."[131] As such, and echoing Paul, it means that God loves *me*. God loves me as a sinner who lives in rebellion against God and all that God loves. God loves me as a sinner—but far too much to leave me as a sinner in a state of rebellion. Instead, God takes *me*—the same me that has turned away from God and God's ways—and God loves me enough to reclaim me and restore me and renew me, and then eventually to perfect me. Now, what is ultimate about me is not, say, identity politics or even personal history. As Eastman says, "When the 'I' is crucified with Christ, the ego is unmoored from any prior sources of identity, worth, direction, or conversely, all sources of shame, dishonor, and despair..."[132] What is of ultimate importance is the fact that I am joined in union with Christ. And, as Chrysostom recognized so long ago, this fact has truly radical consequences for my life, the life I "now live" in "the flesh."

1.6 Conclusion

In this chapter I have offered a theological interpretation of Gal 2:19–20. I have done so in dialogue with the proposals of several leading apocalyptic interpreters. These proposals are intriguing, and I have explored various ways of extending them and possibly strengthening them. My theological analysis has offered some criticisms and raised significant concerns about the radical apocalyptic interpretations. Perhaps those criticisms can be adequately addressed and the concerns alleviated, but I have moved in a different direction. Drawing upon a much older interpretation of the passage—while also receiving with gratitude some insights from the apocalyptic school—I opt for a different account. It is one that is also—in its own way—"radical" indeed. For, if I am right, what we should learn from Paul's teaching is that God's saving work in Christ goes all the way to the "roots" or "core" of our being: those who are joined in union with Christ are truly transformed and sanctified entirely.

If I am joined in union with Christ, then this life—the life that I live *now*, in this *flesh, this* life—is lived by faith in the Son of God, the incarnate Son who loved me and gave himself for me.

---

[131] Wright, *Paul and His Recent Interpreters*, p. 344.
[132] Susan G. Eastman, *Paul and the Person: Reframing Paul's Anthropology* (Grand Rapids: William B. Eerdmans Publishing Co., 2017), p. 174.

2

The Faith of the Son

Pistis Christou Reconsidered

2.1 Introduction

Few disagreements have roiled Pauline scholarship in recent decades (in English-speaking circles) more than the debate over how to understand Paul's references to πίστις Χριστοῦ.[1] The phrase itself occurs seven times in three Pauline letters (Rom 3:22, 26; twice in Gal 2:16; 2:20; 3:22; Phil 3:9). Just what does it mean? How is Paul's phrase to be understood? Everyone understands that Paul employs a genitive construction here, but how is it to be translated and understood? More specifically, is this to be taken as an "objective genitive"—does Paul here refer to human faith *in* Christ? Or is to be understood as a "subjective genitive"—is Paul talking about the faith or faithfulness *of* Christ? And what difference does it make? Just what is at stake theologically in this exegetical debate? In this chapter, I offer theological analysis of some of the more interesting developments in this debate, and I make a modest proposal that draws upon some oft-overlooked and sometimes misunderstood resources from the tradition of scholastic Protestant exegesis and theology.

[1] I say "in English-speaking circles" because the recent debates have mostly involved British, Canadian, and American scholars. James D. G. Dunn reports that an earlier phase of the debate occurred (about a century ago) primarily in German scholarship, "Once More, ΠΙΣΤΙΣ ΧΡΙΣΤΟΥ," reprinted in Richard Hays, *The Faith of Jesus Christ: The Narrative Substructure of Galatians 3:1–4:11*, second edition (Grand Rapids: William B. Eerdmans Publishing Co., 2002), p. 249. See also the summary of the debate's backstory by R. Michael Allen, *The Christ's Faith: A Dogmatic Account* (New York: T&T Clark, 2009), pp. 9–25.

Analytic Christology and the Theological Interpretation of the New Testament. Thomas H. McCall, Oxford University Press (2021). © Thomas H. McCall. DOI: 10.1093/oso/9780198857495.003.0003

2.2 The Current Debate

2.2.1 Faith *in* Christ: The Traditional "Lutheran" Reading

Deeply traditional interpretations of this Pauline phrase are well-known and even intuitive for many Christian readers.[2] When Paul refers to πίστις Χριστου, he refers to faith in Christ. More specifically, he refers to *human* faith in Christ; he is talking about a relationship of belief and trust that somehow is important in bringing about the justification and finally the salvation of sinners. In his letter to the Galatians, Paul says "we know that a person is justified not by the works of the law but through faith *in Jesus Christ*," and "*we* have come to believe in Jesus Christ, so that we might be justified *by faith in Christ*, and not by doing the works of the law" (Gal 2:16). Justification by *human faith* in Jesus Christ is contrasted with justification by *human effort* (the "works of the law"). Beyond justification, Paul exclaims that the "new life" of the redeemed is "lived in the flesh" precisely "by faith *in the Son of God who loved me and gave himself for me*" (Gal 2:20).

This position often wears the label "Lutheran," but, to the extent that it captures traditional views at all, it is obviously much broader than Luther's own theology or even confessional Lutheranism.[3] More commonly, it is called "the anthropological view" or referred to as the *objective* interpretation; anthropological because it refers to the faith of human persons, and "objective" because Jesus Christ is the object of the faith.

Arguments for this position are drawn from a variety of angles and sources. Some of the older arguments for the venerable doctrine are more obviously broadly theological in nature. For instance, as Thomas Aquinas points out, anyone who enjoys the beatific vision does not have faith (as "faith" is biblically defined or depicted). And the incarnate Son surely

---

[2] There is some debate over exactly how broad and deep this interpretation is in the tradition, but no one doubts that it is widespread and deep-seated. Ian G. Wallis argues that the "subjective" interpretation is actually ancient but is then pushed aside by the "objective" interpretations as pro-Nicene theologians in the fourth century (especially Athanasius) are driven by their battles with Arianism and other non-Nicene and anti-Nicene theologies to deny that Christ had faith. See Ian G. Wallis, *The Faith of Jesus Christ in Early Christian Traditions* (Cambridge: Cambridge University Press, 1995), pp. 200–212. For penetrating criticism of Wallis's case, see Mark W. Elliott, "πίστις Χριστου in the Church Fathers and Beyond," in Michael F. Bird and Preston M. Sprinkle, eds., *The Faith of Jesus Christ: Exegetical, Biblical, and Theological Studies* (Peabody: Hendrickson Publishers, 2009), pp. 277–289.

[3] See the observations made by Stephen Westerholm on the label "Lutheran" in contemporary New Testament studies in *Perspectives Old and New on Paul: The "Lutheran" Paul and His Critics* (Grand Rapids: William B. Eerdmans Publishing Co., 2004), p. xvii.

enjoys the beatific vision—even as a wayfarer and, indeed, even during his passion. Thus we can be certain that the Son does not have faith.[4] But such overtly theological considerations are not nearly so common in the recent literature, and in their place we are more likely to find a battery of arguments drawn from linguistic and historical considerations. Thus arguments are made from the use of the definite article, from the relation of faith to the "works of the law," from alternative manuscript traditions, and from Paul's appeal to the faith of Abraham.[5] Exegetes who align with traditional interpretations and influential advocates of the New Perspective on Paul alike continue to hold to the "objective" or "anthropological" position.

2.2.2 The Faith *of* Christ: A Recurring Proposal

During the middle part of the last century, Thomas F. Torrance made the case that we should understand Paul to be talking in the first instance about the faith and faithfulness of Christ.[6] His case relied heavily on an underlying "Hebrew meaning" of the term, and it was soon subjected to blistering criticism from James Barr. In the words of Richard Hays, Barr's onslaught was a "withering critique."[7] The dust-up between Torrance and Barr served to both draw attention to the debate and, for a while at least, to stifle it. But it was bound to re-ignite.

The more recent controversy was kicked into high gear by the publication of Richard Hays's influential work. Hays argues that Torrance was

---

[4] Thomas Aquinas, *Summa Theologica* III.7.3.

[5] On arguments from the use of the definite article, see especially James D. G. Dunn, "Once More, πίστις Χριστοῦ," p. 253; Gordon D. Fee, *Pauline Christology: An Exegetical-Theological Study* (Peabody, Hendrickson, 2007), pp. 224–225; and, more recently, Stanley E. Porter and A. W. Pitts, "πίστις with an Preposition and Genitive Modifier: Lexical, Semantic, and Syntactic Considerations in the πίστις Χριστοῦ Discussion," in Michael F. Bird and Preston M. Sprinkle, eds., *The Faith of Jesus Christ: Exegetical, Biblical, and Theological Studies* (Peabody: Hendrickson Publishers, 2009), pp. 49–51. For arguments that appeal to insights drawn from various manuscript traditions, see especially Barry Matlock, "'Even the Demons Believe': Paul and πίστις Χριστοῦ," *Catholic Biblical Quarterly* 64:2 (2002), pp. 300–318; Matlock, "πίστις in Gal 3:26: Neglected Evidence for Faith in Christ?" *New Testament Studies* 49:3 (2003), pp. 433–439. For consideration of the faith of Abraham, see Dunn, "Once More," pp. 265, 270–271; James D. G. Dunn, "Faith, Faithfulness," in *The New Interpreters Bible Dictionary Vol. 2: D-H* (Nashville: Abingdon Press, 2007), pp. 407–423; and H. Wayne Johnson, "The Paradigm of Abraham in Galatians 3:6-9," *Trinity Journal* 8 (1987), pp. 179–199.

[6] Thomas F. Torrance, "One Aspect of the Biblical Conception of Faith," *Expository Times* 68:4 (1957), pp. 111–114.

[7] Richard Hays, *The Faith of Jesus Christ: The Narrative Substructure of Galatians 3:1–4:11*, second edition (Grand Rapids: William B. Eerdmans Publishing Co., 2002), p. xxxi n23.

fundamentally right—even if Torrance's arguments were vulnerable and his case was weak, nonetheless it turns out that his position was correct. Hays makes a powerful case for the subjective genitive or "Christological" interpretation. He is joined by many luminaries in New Testament scholarship, and together they mount an impressive array of exegetical arguments in favor of their view.[8] Some of the arguments are more grammatical and narrowly contextual; others are more attuned to the broader patterns of Pauline thought more generally. Some defenders of the Christological reading argue that to take Paul's term as an objective genitive (or in the "anthropological" sense) is to posit artificial and needless repetition in some places; Hays argues that the objective genitive reading of Rom 3:22 leaves us with a "peculiar redundancy."[9] Proponents of the subjective or Christological reading argue further that Paul emphatically juxtaposes divine action against human effort; Paul is not at pains to show that the problem is with the wrong kind of human effort—as if all that is needed for salvation is to swap out frenetic efforts to do the right thing in keeping the law for equally frenetic efforts to reach the right cognitive state by believing the correct orthodoxy. Paul's point, in other words, is not to trade one form of human activity for another. Instead Paul is exercised to show the contrast between the bankruptcy of all human striving and the efficacy and power of God's decisive action in Jesus Christ. Thus Hays says that "the whole passage [here Gal 3:2–5] makes better sense if we suppose that Paul's primary intention is not at all to juxtapose one type of human activity ('works') to another ('believing-hearing') but rather to juxtapose human activity to God's activity, as revealed in the 'proclamation.'"[10] Some proponents of this view rely heavily on a particular reading of Hab 2:4 as background.[11] And throughout is an insistence that, for Paul, God's righteousness is revealed by faith—but such divine righteousness is not (and perhaps cannot be) unveiled by human belief (or activity). As Douglas

---

[8] For this summary of the major arguments I am indebted to Matthew C. Easter, "The *Pistis Christou* Debate: Main Arguments and Responses in Summary," *Currents in Biblical Research* 9:1 (2010), pp. 33–47.

[9] Richard Hays, *The Faith of Jesus Christ*, p. 283. Cf. Luke Timothy Johnson, "Romans 3:21–26 and the Faith of Jesus," *Catholic Biblical Quarterly* 44:1 (1982), pp. 77–90; Leander Keck, "'Jesus' in Romans," *Journal of Biblical Literature* 68:3 (1989), pp. 443–460; Frank J. Matera, *Galatians* (Collegeville: Liturgical Press, 1992), pp. 454–456.

[10] Hays, *The Faith of Jesus Christ*, p. 130.

[11] E.g., Hays, *The Faith of Jesus Christ*, pp. 132–141; Douglas A. Campbell, "Romans 1:17 – a Crux Interpretum for the πίστις Χριστοῦ Debate," *Journal of Biblical Literature* 113:2 (1994), pp. 282–284; Douglas A. Campbell, *The Deliverance of God: An Apocalyptic Re-Reading of Justification in Paul* (Grand Rapids: William B. Eerdmans Publishing Co., 2009), pp. 613–616.

Campbell puts it, "Human 'faith' cannot function instrumentally with a process of divine disclosure...Yet these texts speak of disclosure, from the divine realm to the human. Something is progressing from God to the world, and this is by means of 'faith.' Hence Christ, again, is the most obvious reading of this data."[12]

This position is often called the "subjective" interpretation, and sometimes it is referred to as the "Christological" reading. The basic point should be obvious: when Paul refers to πίστις Χριστου, he is talking about the faith had and displayed by Jesus Christ himself. Thus Paul's statements to the Galatians are to be understood as pointing away from human faith and to the reality and soteriological efficacy of Christ's own faith: "we know that a person is justified not by the works of the law but through *the faith of Jesus Christ*" (Gal 2:16), and the life that Paul "now lives in the flesh" he lives "by the faith *of the Son of God*" who lovingly gave himself for Paul (Gal 2:20).

2.2.3 Faith *in and with* Christ: Further Developments

While the "objective" and "subjective" interpretations have attracted the most attention (and the most defenders), not all Pauline scholars are content with those options.[13] Morna D. Hooker notes that "the phrase could convey both meanings simultaneously."[14] Citing Nigel Turner, she reminds us that "grammarians 'warn us against being over precise,' for 'there is no reason why a gen[itive] in the author's mind may not have been both subjective and objective.'"[15] Grammatical analysis allows for the possibility that it is both, and Hooker makes an exegetical and theological case that it is preferable to regard it as both. She suggests that "the answer to the question 'Does this faith refer to Christ's faith or ours?' may be 'Both.' Nevertheless, that faith/faithfulness is primarily that of Christ, and we share in it only because we are in him."[16] So although it is true that the weight of the exegetical evidence

---

[12] Douglas A. Campbell, *The Quest for Paul's Gospel: A Suggested Strategy* (New York: T&T Clark, 2005), p. 197. Cf. Hays, *The Faith of Jesus Christ*, pp. 158–160.

[13] E.g., Preston M. Sprinkle, "Πίστις Χριστου as an Eschatological Event," in Michael F. Bird and Preston M. Sprinkle, eds., *The Faith of Jesus Christ: Exegetical, Biblical, and Theological Studies* (Peabody: Hendrickson Publishers, 2009), pp. 165–184; Jonathan Linebaugh, "The Christo-centrism of Faith in Christ: Martin Luther's Reading of Galatians 2.16, 19-20," *New Testament Studies* 59:4 (2013), pp. 535–544.

[14] Morna D. Hooker, "Another Look at πίστις Χριστου," *Scottish Journal of Theology* 69:1 (2016), p. 48.

[15] Hooker, "Another Look," p. 48.   [16] Hooker, "Another Look," p. 62.

favors the traditional, "Lutheran," objective (or "anthropological") position, nonetheless "it would seem that this faith is possible only because it is a sharing in his."[17] Thus she concludes that "in Christ, and through him, we are able to share his trust and obedience, and so become what God called his people to be."[18]

2.2.4 Moving Forward: The Inevitability of Theological Interpretation

It is important to note that the issues are complex at several levels. As we have seen, the meaning of the genitive is a point of discussion and debate. But the term often translated *faith* is also ambiguous; it may mean something more like belief or trust (or both), but it could also mean something more like faithfulness.[19] In other words, it might be referring to something closer to epistemology, or it might be referencing something more like ethics. The major options for understanding πίστις Χριστου could be construed as:

(α) human belief and trust in Jesus Christ;
(β) believing and faithful human obedience to Jesus Christ;
(γ) the trusting belief of Jesus Christ;
(δ) the trusting and faithful obedience of Jesus Christ.

Just what are we to make of all this? What is at stake? And how might this debate be settled? Advocates of the major interpretative camps often recognize that the more narrowly exegetical (grammatical and historical) considerations are not finally decisive in these debates. Thus Hays, while standing by his "earlier judgment that the balance of grammatical evidence strongly favors the subjective genitive interpretation and that the arguments for an objective genitive are fairly weak," nonetheless understands that "such syntactical arguments are, however, finally inconclusive."[20] Hooker's verdict is decisive: "the appeal to grammar has, in effect, run into the sand."[21] Such

---

[17] Hooker, "Another Look," p. 62.   [18] Hooker, "Another Look," p. 62.
[19] Additionally, it might be used as shorthand for the content of belief; as Hooker puts it, "what one believes," "Another Look," p. 48.
[20] Hays, *The Faith of Jesus Christ*, p. 276.
[21] Hooker, "Another Look," p. 46. On the other hand, Stanley E. Porter and Andrew W. Pitts argue that "lexical, grammatical, and syntactical factors are probably more important to the

an admission does not, however, mean that it is impossible to make cogent arguments or otherwise to make progress in these discussions. But what such an admission does mean is that further considerations will be overtly theological in nature. To quote Hays again, further arguments "must be governed by larger judgments about the shape and logic of Paul's thought concerning faith, Christ, and salvation."[22] Debbie Hunn is even more blunt: "It is theology, not grammar, that continues to drive the debate."[23]

Indeed, even what appears at first glance to be a more "exegetical" argument actually is seen, upon closer consideration, to rely upon distinctly theological considerations. As an example, consider Douglas Campbell's argument (in favor of the subjective or Christological interpretation) from Paul's convictions about the unveiling of righteousness (in Rom 3:21–22). Campbell insists that

> Human "faith" cannot function instrumentally within a process of divine disclosure. This is semantically impossible. "Faith" does not function actually to disclose information; it does not make something that is invisible visible. This is not what it means or denotes. Yet these texts speak of disclosure... Hence Christ, again, is the most obvious reading of this data.[24]

But why? Is this so obvious? Given various theological assumptions (especially those of the "apocalyptic" school), Campbell's point may seem indisputable. Without those assumptions, however, the point is not so secure. His argument is that human faith or faithfulness cannot reveal anything true of God. Faith is a response to divine revelation; it is not revelation itself or even the vehicle of it. So faith cannot be revelatory; it does not "disclose information" or "make something that is invisible visible."

---

discussion than is usually assumed," "Πίστις with a Preposition and Genitive Modifier: Lexical, Semantic, and Syntactical Considerations in the πίστις Χριστου Discussion," in Michael F. Bird and Preston M. Sprinkle, eds., *The Faith of Jesus Christ: Exegetical, Biblical, and Theological Studies* (Peabody: Hendrickson Publishers, 2009), p. 36.

[22] Hays, *The Faith of Jesus Christ*, p. 277.

[23] Debbie Hunn, "Debating the Faithfulness of Jesus Christ in Twentieth Century Scholarship," in Michael F. Bird and Preston M. Sprinkle, eds., *The Faith of Jesus Christ: Exegetical, Biblical, and Theological Studies* (Peabody: Hendrickson Publishers, 2009), p. 26.

[24] Douglas A. Campbell, *The Quest for Paul's Gospel: A Suggested Strategy* (London: T&T Clark, 2005), p. 197.

But, again, why not? Consider someone who has only ever heard talk about justice or righteousness or faith. For the person who has never seen it, such talk may be exciting and foreign. *Sans* enactment, however, such talk may also be impossibly vague, and at any rate sound only like an eschatological pipe dream. But now consider someone who sees it enacted and lived out. Would there not be a sense in which this "makes something that is invisible visible"—would not a lived and embodied practice of faithful righteousness actually "disclose information" that is important (i.e., lived and embodied faithful righteousness is not only possible but also indeed actual)? Indeed, is this not something close to what is depicted in the famous statements about faith in Hebrews 11–12 (where Christ is ultimate but the other runners who have finished the course are also both exemplars and encouragers)? Perhaps Campbell's central concern is one about the primacy and prevenience of divine agency; maybe he is only exercised to insist that any authentic claims to knowledge of God can only be made in response to divine grace rather than productive of that grace. If so, then his point is well-taken and always appropriate. But if so, then it is also hard to see how it supports his conclusion that human faith cannot reveal what is divine. Moreover, as it stands, Campbell claims too much. He denies that *human* faith can "function instrumentally" in divine revelation. But as it stands, such a claim will be problematic for his own view. Is not this exactly what the incarnate divine Son does (on Campbell's "apocalyptic" theology as much as any other)? As it stands, his statement excludes the possibility of divine revelation in the incarnation of the Son. Presumably, when Campbell speaks in this context of "human faith," he refers to the faith of one who is *merely human* rather than *truly human*. But this could be usefully clarified, especially if it is meant to serve as a defeater for the traditional position.

At any rate, we have now arrived at a place in which the inevitability of theological interpretation is recognized. We are also dealing with an issue that is widely understood to be theologically pregnant and indeed very important. As Hays recognizes, "there are serious theological issues at stake here."[25] So, once again, just what *are* those issues? Just what is at stake theologically? Hays identifies several theological issues, some of which are of critical importance. First, we see that these discussions have implications for an adequate account of theology proper. Immediately, Hays has in mind a correct understanding of the righteousness of God as

---

[25] Hays, *The Faith of Jesus Christ*, p. 292.

"covenant-faithfulness," but the concerns extend further.[26] Hays wants to develop a proper relationship between the covenant-faithfulness of God and the divine attributes more broadly. A second area of theological concern has to do with the humanity of Jesus. Hays is worried about "implicitly docetic Christology."[27] Third, and closely related, are matters of Christology and soteriology. Such soteriological concerns include the very basis of the human hope of salvation: are sinners saved by their own efforts to believe the right concepts, or are they saved by the faithfulness *of Christ*?[28] Finally, and closely related, we encounter ethical concerns: how are we to account for the straightforward Pauline ethical admonitions and exhortations to live "the same sort of faith-obedience that he revealed?"[29]

2.3 The *Πίστις Χριστου* Debate and the Humanity of Christ

As we have seen, Hays is concerned about the humanity of Christ. So let us consider this worry. Recall Hays's concern to affirm the full and authentic humanity of Christ. Hays says that "some opposition to the Christological interpretation may be rooted in an implicitly docetic Christology. If Jesus was a real human being, it is hardly scandalous or inappropriate to speak of his faith/fidelity toward God."[30] Note that Hays says only that *some* opposition to the Christological reading *may* stem from docetism. He does not say that such opposition necessarily does or even that it always does. He only indicates that docetism may be a factor that militates against the Christological reading. Taken as such—as a general worry about what *may* motivate *some* forms of opposition—the concern of Hays should not be controversial. To the contrary, it may be a word in season.

But it would be a mistake to extend what Hays says into a broader critique of the anthropological interpretation more generally. There is nothing about the anthropological interpretation that is obviously docetic, and it is not easy to see how an argument for this conclusion might be made successfully.

---

[26] Hays, *The Faith of Jesus Christ*, p. 294.   [27] Hays, *The Faith of Jesus Christ*, p. 293.
[28] As Chris Tilling notes, "The key issue for Campbell is that faith is *not* to be understood, as the theoretical logic of a conventional reading of Romans 1–4 arguably demands, as the *condition* of salvation," although it nonetheless somehow is "necessary if final life or salvation is to be reached," "Campbell's Faith: Advancing the *Pistis Christou* Debate," in Chris Tilling, ed., *Beyond Old and New Perspectives on Paul: Reflections on the Work of Douglas Campbell* (Eugene: Cascade Books, 2014), p. 237.
[29] Hays, *The Faith of Jesus Christ*, p. 294.   [30] Hays, *The Faith of Jesus Christ*, p. 293.

Consider the position of Aquinas. He is certain that Christ does not possess faith, and he is confident of this because he is sure that Christ has the beatific vision during his days as an earthly sojourner. Faith has to do with those things that are true of God that are "not seen" (Heb 11:1). But since Christ has the beatific vision, then there is nothing that is "not seen." Thus Christ does not, strictly speaking, have faith. Would this mean that Aquinas's doctrine is docetic? Not at all. Unless we have good reason to think that possession of the beatific vision is not possible for someone who is human (or, perhaps, for someone who is an *embodied* human), then there is no reason to conclude that Christ (or anyone else) would have had to have faith in order to be human. But we do not have such reasons. Moreover, while the relation of the incarnate Christ to the beatific vision in his wayfaring days may be the subject of disagreement, it is hardly controversial among theologians to hold that the incarnate Christ enjoys the beatific vision during his ascension and session—which is to say, *now*. Yet Christ surely remains human throughout the ascension and session, so being human is not incompossible with the beatific vision. According to the very traditional theology that adamantly rejects docetism, Christ enjoys the beatific vision as fully human—and, indeed, so shall all human persons who are joined in union with Christ in the eschaton.

2.4 *Πίστις Χριστου* and the Righteousness of God

2.4.1 Hays on the Christological Revelation of the Divine Attributes

In his illuminating study of Paul's use of Scripture, Hays says that the "keynote of Paul's exposition sounds in Rom. 1:16–17: 'I am not ashamed of the gospel, for it is the power of God for salvation [*soterion*] to everyone who believes, to the Jew first but also to the Greek. For through the gospel the righteousness of God [*dikaiosyne theou*] is revealed [*apokalyptetai*], from faith for faith, just as it is written, 'The righteous one shall live from faith.'"[31] Hays notes the resonance with key passages from the LXX. Psalm 97:2 says that "The Lord has made known his salvation [*soterion*]; in the presence of the nations [*ethnon*] he has revealed [*apekalypsen*] his

---

[31] Richard B. Hays, *Echoes of Scripture in the Letters of Paul* (New Haven: Yale University Press, 1989), p. 36.

righteousness [*dikaiosynen*]."[32] Hays sees this as a sharp summary of Paul's account of the good news: God's righteousness is unveiled and displayed in what God has done in Jesus Christ, and this righteousness is revealed as nothing other than God's faithfulness. According to the prophets, God's plan of salvation is meant for both Jews and Gentiles. Thus we read in Isaiah that God's justice will be a light to the Gentiles, and God says that "my righteousness [*dikaiosyne*] draws near quickly, and my salvation [*soterion*] will go forth as a light, and in my arm [cf. *dynamis* in Rom 1:16] will Gentiles [*ethne*] hope" (Isa. 51:4–5).[33] Moreover, "the Lord will reveal [*apokalypsei*] his holy arm before all the Gentiles [*ethnon*], and all the corners of the earth will see the salvation [*soterion*] that is with God" (Isa. 52:10).[34] When Paul says "I am not ashamed," he is echoing the psalms and prophets (cf. Ps 43:10 LXX; 24:2 LXX; Isa 28:16 LXX).[35] But there is an important change: for "Paul transforms Isaiah's emphatic future negation ('I shall not be ashamed') into a present negation ('I *am* not ashamed'). The present tense of Paul's denial corresponds to the present tense of his declaration that the righteousness and wrath of God *are being* revealed (1:17–18); thus Isaiah's future hope rebounds through Paul's voice into a new temporal framework defined by God's already efficacious act of eschatological deliverance in Christ."[36]

Hays argues that Paul builds this case as Romans progresses: Paul is not ashamed of this gospel of God that has been intended for all and that has now come to all in the person of Jesus Christ. What the gospel revealed in Christ shows is that "God's truthfulness (*aletheia*, cf. Rom 3:4–7) and righteousness (*dikaiosyne*, cf. Rom 3:5, 21–22)" is the "ground of hope and instrument of deliverance."[37] Closely echoing Psalm 143, Paul's teaching is that divine righteousness is "a witness concerning God's gracious saving power . . ."[38] For God "has put forward Jesus Christ as an 'indication of his righteousness' [*endeixin tes dikaiosynes autou*]" (Rom 3:25–26). And God has done this "in order that he [God] might himself be righteousness even in justifying the person who lives through the faithfulness of Jesus."[39]

With this background in mind, let us return to the Christological considerations. Hays notes "some positive correlation between the christological ('subjective genitive') construal and an affirmation of the centrality of Israel/

[32] Hays, *Echoes of Scripture*, p. 36. The reference in the Masoretic Text is to 98:2.
[33] Hays, *Echoes of Scripture*, p. 37.   [34] Hays, *Echoes of Scripture*, p. 37.
[35] See the discussion in Hays, *Echoes of Scripture*, pp. 38–39.
[36] Hays, *Echoes of Scripture*, p. 39.   [37] Hays, *Echoes of Scripture*, p. 52.
[38] Hays, *Echoes of Scripture*, p. 52.   [39] Hays, *Echoes of Scripture*, p. 53.

covenant themes in Paul's theology."[40] The "key," he says, is to "recognize that Paul's defense of God's faithfulness to Israel in Romans 3:3–5 (ἡ πίστις του θεο = θεου δικαιοσύνη) is linked to his affirmation that the righteousness of God (δικαιοσύνη θεου) has been manifested through the faithfulness of Jesus Christ (διὰ πίστεως Ιησου Χριστου 3:21–22)."[41] Hays is well aware that the connection here is less than straightforward, and he recognizes that the issues are complicated. He notes, for instance, that he is in agreement with Dunn but very much opposed to J. Louis Martyn in holding that the righteousness of God is to be equated with God's covenant faithfulness— but opposed to Dunn and in agreement with Martyn on the meaning of πίστις Χριστου.[42] So "a theological judgment" about divine righteousness "is not strictly tied to one's exegetical decision about πίστις Χριστου," but surely it is closely related, and "further analysis" would do well to sort these matters out further.[43]

But what does such "further analysis" show? So far as I can see, it shows that the Christological or subjective genitive reading is not sufficient for the conclusion that we should equate divine righteousness with covenant faithfulness. As Hays recognizes, scholars with different views of πίστις Χριστου come to varying conclusions about the relationship of righteousness to covenant faithfulness. It is less than obvious that they flaunt coherence in doing so. So having the "right" view of πίστις Χριστου does not guarantee the "right" stance on divine righteousness.

But theological analysis also shows that the Christological or subjective genitive reading is not necessary to link divine righteousness very closely to covenant faithfulness (and perhaps even to equate them). Hays wants to hold together very closely what he refers to as "three apparently synonymous attributes of God": ἡ πίστις του θεου, θεου δικαιοσύνη, ἡ ἀλήθεια του θεου "(the faithfulness of God, God's righteousness, and the truthfulness of God)".[44] I take it that Hays wants to avoid any suggestion that divine righteousness and justice and faithfulness are somehow arbitrary to God, or that divine righteousness might be essential to God—but God's covenant faithfulness and truthfulness are somehow arbitrary. And, of course, he wants to maintain the conviction that these divine attributes are truly revealed by Jesus Christ. There is good news for Hays: as it turns out, there is more than one way to hold these attributes together very closely,

[40] Hays, *The Faith of Jesus Christ*, p. 294.   [41] Hays, *The Faith of Jesus Christ*, p. 294.
[42] Hays, *The Faith of Jesus Christ*, p. 294.   [43] Hays, *The Faith of Jesus Christ*, p. 294.
[44] Hays, *The Faith of Jesus Christ*, p. 282.

and they allow us to do so in ways that keeps Christ at the center of the revelation. As it also turns out, none of these ways requires a decision between the subjective and objective interpretations.

2.4.2 Keeping It Simple: *Ressourcing* Traditional Doctrines of God

Consider what happens to Hays's desiderata if one accepts the venerable doctrine of divine simplicity. On simplicity, these are not merely "apparently synonymous attributes." For, on simplicity, there is no "real distinction" between the divine attributes at all. According to the doctrine of divine simplicity, God is not composed or built up out of parts or pieces. So while it is, of course, appropriate and fitting for us to refer to various divine attributes, we should never be misled by our language into thinking that God is somehow really made up of distinct components or parts. On "Thomist" doctrines of simplicity, the distinctions between the divine attributes are only "rational" or conceptual, and while it is appropriate to refer to them as distinct, this manner of speaking tells us more about our relation to God than it does about any real distinctions in God (much like it is entirely appropriate to refer to the "morning star" and the "evening star" even while we realize that they aren't two different "things").[45] Or on "Scotist" accounts of the doctrine, the "formal distinction" lies between merely rational or conceptual distinctions, on one hand, and "real" distinctions, on the other.[46] Where "real" distinctions are distinctions between different things (either things of the same essence or different things of different essences) or between separable parts of the same thing, entities that are formally distinct are genuinely but not "really" distinct (again, where a "real" distinction picks out separable entities). On broadly Scotist doctrines of simplicity, the divine attributes are not independent things that could exist on their own, but nor

---

[45] For a summary account of Thomas Aquinas's doctrine of divine simplicity, see Eleonore Stump, *Aquinas* (New York: Routledge, 2003), pp. 92–130. On the reception of traditional accounts in Protestant scholasticism, see Richard A. Muller, *Post-Reformation Reformed Dogmatics: The Rise and Development of Reformed Orthodoxy, ca. 1520 to ca. 1725, Volume Three: The Divine Essence and Attributes* (Grand Rapids: Baker Academic, 2003), pp. 38–44, 53–58, 275–298; and Steven J. Duby, *Divine Simplicity: A Dogmatic Account*, T&T Clark Studies in Systematic Theology (New York: Bloomsbury T&T Clark, 2016), pp. 18–25.

[46] For a helpful account of John Duns Scotus's doctrine, see Richard Cross, *Duns Scotus on God* (Aldershot: Ashgate, 2005), pp. 99–114. On closely related issues in metaphysics, see Mary Beth Ingham and Mechthild Dreyer, *The Philosophical Vision of John Duns Scotus* (Washington: The Catholic University of America Press, 2004), pp. 33–51.

are they identical. Instead, the divine attributes are genuinely distinct but not even possibly independent. Either way, whether one opts for Thomist or Scotist versions of the doctrine, the payoff is the same: one can have a very strong connection between various divine attributes without relying upon an exegetical conclusion that is hotly contested.

2.4.3 Making It Complex: Contemporary Essentialism and the Doctrine of God

A critic might point out, however, that such doctrines of simplicity are themselves hotly contested. Fair enough. But one need not go all the way to a "Thomist" or even "Scotist" account to see how theological analysis that yields a more modest version of the doctrine might still be of assistance to someone who shares the convictions of Hays. Recent work in analytic metaphysics and theology provides resources to think constructively about the relation of divine righteousness to divine faithfulness (as well as divine truthfulness).

Because this discussion will assume the use of recent developments in the metaphysics of modality, perhaps it will help to briefly summarize the relevant operative concepts. First, in what follows I assume that reality has a modal structure, and further that the system of modal logic known as S5 is the best option available to us.[47] "Modal logic" in this context simply refers to the conceptual tools that have been developed to help us think better about terms that enjoy everyday and intuitive usage; I refer here to terms such as *possibly, necessarily, might have, could have, could not have, would have*, and *would not have*. S5 is widely considered to be the most advanced and most complete system available, and it is often understood to include or contain the insights of the other systems.[48] The characteristic axiom is *if possibly p, then necessarily possibly p.*[49] To this we add the concept of possible worlds. A possible world is a state of affairs; more precisely, it is a maximally consistent state of affairs.[50] Employing S5 with possible worlds

---

[47] I include here De Morgan equivalences ($\Diamond{\sim}p \Longleftrightarrow {\sim}\Box p$ and ${\sim}\Diamond p \Longleftrightarrow \Box{\sim}p$) as well as the Distribution Axiom (if ($\Box p \Rightarrow q$), then $\Box p \Rightarrow \Box q$). For a recent helpful overview, see Alexander R. Pruss and Joshua L. Rasmussen, *Necessary Existence* (Oxford: Oxford University Press, 2018), pp. 14–15.

[48] Especially T ($\Box p \Rightarrow p$), the *Brouweresche* ($p \Rightarrow \Box\Diamond p$), and S4 ($\Box p \Rightarrow \Box\Box p$).

[49] ($\Diamond p \Rightarrow \Box\Diamond p$).

[50] See Alvin Plantinga, *The Nature of Necessity* (Oxford: Oxford University Press, 1974), pp. 44–45.

semantics brings us to essentialism.[51] As Plantinga explains, "an object has a property *essentially* if it has it in such a way that it is not even possible that it exist but *fail* to have it."[52] To account for temporality, we might follow E. J. Lowe: "an essential property of an object is a property which that object always possesses and which it could not have failed to possess—in other words, in the language of possible worlds, it is a property which that object possesses at all times in every possible world."[53] Accordingly, when we turn our attention to consideration of the divine essence and attributes, essential divine attributes are those that are possessed by God in every possible world in which God exists. So, if God exists necessarily (in every possible world), then essential divine attributes are those that God has in all possible worlds. (Alternatively, if God exists only "contingently" rather than necessarily, then essential divine attributes are those that God possesses in all possible worlds in which God has existence.[54])

Now it may seem at first glance that this brief excursus into the metaphysics of modality is very far removed from the exegetical debate over the proper interpretation of pistis christou, and even a long way from Hays's concerns about the relation of divine faithfulness to divine righteousness. But first glances can be misleading, for with these resources it is possible to make several theological affirmations that hold promise for satisfying Hays's concerns about the divine attributes. In fact, there are multiple ways of holding these divine attributes together. Here are three possible ways of doing so.

---

[51] Alvin Plantinga observes that although logical positivism rejected the notions of essences and essential properties as not only outdated but also incoherent, "Through a delicious historical irony, however, essences and essentialism received a new lease on life partly through the efforts of the logical positivists. The positivists very commendably emphasized the importance of logic for philosophy; by virtue of this emphasis there arose a renewed interest in modal logic and the semantics of modal logic; and it is but a short step from the semantics of modal logic to an appreciation of the notions of essential properties and essences," "Essence and Essentialism," in Jaegwon Kim and Ernest Sosa, eds., *A Companion to Metaphysics* (Oxford: Blackwell, 1995), p. 139. For an excellent introduction to the renaissance of interest in and defense of essentialism in recent analytic philosophy (and, more specifically, the move from modal logic to the metaphysics of modality), see Michael J. Loux, "Introduction: Modality and Metaphysics," in Michael J. Loux, ed., *The Possible and the Actual* (Ithaca: Cornell University Press, 1979), pp. 15–64. Major works include Alvin Plantinga, *The Nature of Necessity*; David Wiggins, *Sameness and Substance* (Oxford: Blackwell, 1980); and Saul Kripke, *Naming and Necessity* (Cambridge: Harvard University Press, 1972).

[52] Plantinga, "Essence and Essentialism," p. 138.

[53] E. J. Lowe, *A Survey of Metaphysics* (Oxford: Oxford University Press, 2002), p. 96.

[54] See Keith E. Yandell, "Divine Necessity and Divine Goodness," in Thomas V. Morris, ed., *Divine and Human Action: Essays in the Metaphysics of Theism* (Ithaca: Cornell University Press, 1988), pp. 313–344.

First, one might posit that both θεου δικαιοσύνη and ἡ πίστις του θεου are essential divine attributes. Both righteous justice and covenant faithfulness are essential to God. These attributes are necessary for God, and God has them with *de re* necessity. There are no possible worlds in which God exists in which God does not exemplify these attributes. So, assuming that God exists necessarily and thus in all possible worlds, then we can conclude that God exemplifies these attributes in all possible worlds. Accordingly, it is not possible that God does not have these attributes, and thus it is impossible for God to act in any way that is inconsistent with righteous justice and covenant faithfulness. Even though these attributes may not be identical in God, they are nonetheless coextensive in God's own being. Turning to Christology, we can affirm that the covenant faithfulness that Christ exhibits may not be, strictly speaking, identical to the righteous justice of God, but both this righteous justice and this covenant faithfulness are essential to him in virtue of his divinity. It is not possible that he act in any way that is inconsistent with this righteous justice and covenant faithfulness. And we are then to understand Christ's own expression of this righteousness and faithfulness not as an exception to how God acts but as the unveiling of God.

Some theologians may worry that this seems like a category mistake. Is it really right to say that *righteousness* and *justice* belong to God's inner life? As Nicholas Wolterstorff expresses the worry, "How dare one even think of justice in the Trinity? Love is what resides in the Trinity. Love casts out justice."[55] If we think of justice as "meting out" justice, of "pronouncing and executing justice" on wrongdoers, then of course we should not think of justice within the Triune life of God.[56] Things are no better if we expand the concept of justice to think of it in terms of "rendering judgment," where that action involves making decisions where there is conflict and then determining and declaring relative guilt and innocence as well as "meting out" judgment. "No rendering of judgment can occur within the Trinity because neither wrongdoing or conflict occurs within the Trinity."[57] But Wolterstorff argues that the worry is misplaced. He draws an important distinction between what he calls "primary justice" and "secondary justice." "Secondary justice" is the umbrella term for the ways that we commonly conceive of justice; it is justice exercised as retributive or corrective or

---

[55] Nicholas Wolterstorff, "Is There Justice in the Trinity?" in Miroslav Volf and Michael Welker, eds., *God's Life in Trinity* (Minneapolis: Fortress Press, 2006), p. 177.

[56] Wolterstorff, "Is There Justice in the Trinity," p. 177.

[57] Wolterstorff, "Is There Justice in the Trinity," p. 177.

restorative. But secondary justice cannot be ultimate in our conceptions of justice. Wolterstorff argues that secondary justice is only derivative; something is wrong because something is right, and what is wrong is wrong because it fails to match the standard of rightness or righteousness. As such, it must be treated accordingly, and justice is "meted out" accordingly. But when justice is "meted out," it is not ultimate but always secondary. "Primary justice," on the other hand, is treating the other with due respect for the worth of the other. Barring some version of pantheism or panentheism, it is hard to see how secondary justice might properly be attributed to God as an essential property—surely retributive justice is not the kind of thing that characterizes the life of the Triune God *ad intra*; surely it isn't true that God exercises retributive justice in all possible worlds. Wolterstorff, however, argues that secondary justice is actually based on primary justice. And while secondary justice may not be appropriately predicated of the essence of God, surely it is right and proper to say that primary justice is true of the Triune God "on the inside" and indeed necessarily. Wolterstoff's answer is clear and strong: "How could there not be justice within the Trinity . . . How could the members of the Trinity fail to treat each other with due respect for their worth?"[58] Indeed, "not only is there justice in the relation of the persons of the Trinity to each other, justice in their relationship is caught up within love for each other. Justice within the Trinity is not a social relationship within the Trinity in addition to love within the Trinity. Justice in the Trinity is a constituent of love within the Trinity."[59] Properly understood, then, it is appropriate and fitting to predicate δικαιοσύνη of the essence of God. For God is righteous and just in all possible worlds; not only is it true that there are no possible worlds in which God is *un*righteous and *un*just, it is also true that there are no possible worlds where God lacks this attribute.

But even if it is acceptable to predicate righteous justice of the Trinity *ad intra*, how are we to attribute covenant faithfulness to the inner life of God? To be sure, various theologians have pushed back hard against any suggestions that there is anything like an intra-Trinitarian covenant. Karl Barth, for example, says that such a notion is "mythology," for it posits not only multiple divine subjects and thus is open to charges of polytheism but even multiple *legal* subjects and thus introduces a contractual form of legalism

---

into the divine life.[60] So, if we hold the view that covenant faithfulness is essential to God, then we seem to be caught on the horns of a dilemma. Either there is some sort of covenant within the inner life of God, or God necessarily exists in relation to creatures with whom God is related by covenant. The first horn is said to lead to a kind of polytheism, while the second seems to lead toward pantheism or panentheism. The issues are complex and the discussions are complicated, but a theologian could attempt to avoid the first horn by adopting either a version of "Social Trinitarianism" (ST) or some form of "Relative Trinitarianism" (RT). According to ST, the divine persons are "distinct centers of consciousness," and the "Holy Trinity is a divine, transcendent society or community of three fully personal and fully divine entities: the Father, the Son, and the Holy Spirit or Paraclete" who are "wonderfully united by their common divinity, that is, by the possession of the whole generic divine essence" as well as by their "joint redemptive purpose, revelation, and work."[61] Clearly, on ST the divine persons are really distinct and related in mutual love, and it would not be a stretch to think of this love as including faithfulness. But ST may not be the only way forward. For on Peter van Inwagen's version of RT, the divine persons are also to be understood as "those things to which personal pronouns are applicable: a person can use the word 'I' and be addressed as a 'thou'... [and] it is evident that the Persons of the Trinity *are* in this sense 'persons,' *are* someones..."[62] Both ST and RT remain controversial. ST is often charged with tending toward tritheism.[63] RT faces challenges that on other fronts.[64] The debates will surely continue. But there are at least two potential ways out of the problem.

---

[60] Karl Barth, *Church Dogmatics* IV/1, trans. G. W. Bromiley, eds., G. W. Bromiley and T. F. Torrance (Edinburgh: T&T Clark, 1956), p. 65.

[61] Cornelius Plantinga, Jr., "Social Trinity and Tritheism," in Ronald J. Feenstra and Cornelius Plantinga, Jr., eds., *Trinity, Incarnation, and Atonement: Philosophical and Theological Essays* (Notre Dame: University of Notre Dame Press, 1989), pp. 22, 27–28.

[62] Peter van Inwagen, *God, Knowledge, and Mystery: Essays in Philosophical Theology* (Ithaca: Cornell University Press, 1995), pp. 264–265.

[63] E.g., Brian Leftow, "Anti Social Trinitarianism," in Thomas McCall and Michael C. Rea, eds., *Philosophical and Theological Essays on the Trinity* (Oxford: Oxford University Press, 2009), pp. 52–88. See further the debate in *Philosophical and Theological Essays on the Trinity*, pp. 89–168 (with essays by William Lane Craig, Daniel Howard-Snyder, Carl Mosser, and Keith E. Yandell); Thomas H. McCall, *Which Trinity? Whose Monotheism? Philosophical and Systematic Theologians on the Metaphysics of Trinitarian Theology* (Grand Rapids: William B. Eerdmans Publishing Co., 2009), pp. 11–124; William Hasker, *Metaphysics and the Tri-Personal God*, Oxford Studies in Analytic Theology, eds., Michael C. Rea and Oliver D. Crisp (Oxford: Oxford University Press, 2013).

[64] E.g., Michael C. Rea, "Relative Identity and the Doctrine of the Trinity," in Thomas McCall and Michael C. Rea, eds., *Philosophical and Theological Essays on the Trinity* (Oxford: Oxford

A second way of thinking about these matters might be more attractive to those who remain concerned about the specter of tritheism (or, for those who would take the other horn, panentheism). We might hold that righteousness and justice are essential to God while also maintaining that God's covenant faithfulness is the non-essential (and thus non-necessary) expression of the righteousness of God. On this model, righteous justice is essential to God; God has this attribute with *de re* necessity, and there are no possible worlds in which God does not have righteous justice. Existing necessarily, God has this attribute in all possible worlds. God's covenant faithfulness, however, is something that is of a different order. It is not, strictly speaking, essential to God; it is not something that God has in all possible worlds. It may be said to be in some sense grounded in, and issuing from, God's righteous justice, and it is always consistent with God's righteous justice. We could say that God has covenant faithfulness in all possible worlds in which God enacts a covenant. Covenant faithfulness is not something arbitrary for God. It is not something that God has that God could surrender or reject or lose. There are no possible worlds in which God makes a covenant but then fails to act to keep it. There are no possible worlds in which God makes a covenant but then is not faithful to it. Turning again to Christology, when Jesus acts in covenant faithfulness he is revealing how God's righteous justice is displayed and enacted in relationship with creatures—in the πίστις Χριστου passages, with creatures who are sinful and rebellious and broken and hopeless. What Jesus is doing in keeping and fulfilling the covenant is what God is doing, and what Jesus is doing is in no sense an exception or aberration but instead is the unveiling of the righteous justice that is essential to God's own life. "*As I live*," declares YHWH, "I take no pleasure in the death of the wicked" (Ezek 33:11). *As I live*.

A third option awaits those who are more inclined to hew closer to traditional lines (but without a return to scholastic doctrines of divine simplicity). One might hold that, strictly speaking, neither the righteous justice nor the covenant faithfulness of God are essential to God. Neither are true of the divine life "on the inside," for neither accurately characterizes the immanent Trinity. There are possible worlds in which God exists

University Press, 2009), pp. 249–262. For another application of the logic of relative identity to the Trinity, see Jeffrey E. Brower and Michael C. Rea, "Material Constitution and the Trinity," in Thomas McCall and Michael C. Rea, eds., *Philosophical and Theological Essays on the Trinity* (Oxford: Oxford University Press, 2009), pp. 263–282.

but where there is no righteous justice or covenant faithfulness. But this need not lead to the conclusion that either righteousness or faithfulness are arbitrary. For on this account, what is said to be essential to God—what is truly predicated of God in all possible worlds—is the *goodness* of God. On this account, God is good in all possible worlds. As Richard Allen says, God *is* "infinite goodness."[65] And both righteous justice and covenant faithfulness are the expression of that goodness in relation to creation and to creatures. Accordingly, God is righteous and just in relation to God's creatures, and it is not so much as possible for God to be anything but righteous or just in relation to creatures.

Turning again to Christology, what Jesus reveals is the unrelenting and unchanging character of God. Jesus unveils and displays God's righteous justice. Jesus reveals the steadfast and loyal faithfulness of God. What Jesus reveals is not in any sense an aberration or exception to the divine character and life. Instead it is the expression of the nature or character of the Triune God in relation to creatures who are desperate for loyalty and love—and indeed hopeless without it. We can say the following: in all possible worlds, mutual love is shared between the divine persons; there is no possible world in which God is not essentially loving. Love is of the essence of the triune God; God's own being is the life of love given and received between Father, Son, and Holy Spirit. Creation is a contingent action of the triune God, for while God does not in any sense need to create in order to love, nonetheless love is the motivation for God's creative activity and the *telos* or end toward which creation is aimed. There are possible worlds in which there is no realm of created reality, but there are no possible worlds in which God is not love. In all possible worlds, the love of God is *holy* in the sense of being pure and unalloyed. In the possible world that is the actual world, of course there is sin and *unholiness*. Through the means of covenant, God has revealed that God is a holy God and thus that God's love is a holy love. And by the covenant, God is bound to God's people in holy love. Accordingly, there is a sense in which it is not so much as possible that God breaks this covenant, for God's own life is now bound up with it. As God exists necessarily and cannot not exist (at least on mainstream or "Anselmian" versions), then it

---

[65] Richard Allen, *The Life, Experience, and Gospel Labors of Rt. Rev. Richard Allen: To Which is Annexed the Rise and Progress of the African Methodist Episcopal Church in the United States of America, Containing a Narrative of the Yellow Fever in the Year of Our Lord 1793, with an Address to the People of Color in the United States* (Philadelphia: Ford and Ripley, 1880), p. 30.

simply is not possible that this covenant—though made contingently—
might be broken by God.

2.4.4 Summary

Where does this leave us? With multiple ways to keep divine *dik-* and divine
pistis together, and with Christ at the center as the one who ultimately
reveals and displays these truths about God. In other words, Hay's desiderata may be satisfied in various ways, and a theologian need not adopt the
subjective or Christological interpretation to do so. Theological analysis
helps us to see this.

2.5 *Πίστις Χριστου* and Salvation

2.5.1 Hays's Concerns

As we have seen, Hays raises concerns about the relation of Christology to
soteriology. At one level, he is trying to understand how it is that the death of
Christ is the "source of salvation."[66] Hays thinks that there is a "puzzling
arbitrariness" about the relation between Christology and the doctrine of
justification in "standard Lutheran-Reformation accounts of justification by
faith."[67] While he is quick to admit that the subjective genitive interpretation
does not provide him with a "satisfactory elucidation of this mystery," Hays
nonetheless is convinced that his preferred take is "more promising."[68] He
follows Sam Williams in this summary: "Christians are justified by that faith
which derives its very character from [Jesus's] self-giving obedience, that
faith which was first his and has now become theirs."[69]

At another and related level, Hays is concerned to properly understand
the "cruciform character of Christian obedience."[70] As he sees matters,
the subjective genitive or Christological interpretation "has the effect of
stressing the pattern of correspondence between Jesus and the believing
community: those who are in Christ are called to live the same sort of
faith-obedience that he revealed."[71] Thus, from a "theological point of

[66] Hays, *The Faith of Jesus Christ*, p. 293.
[67] Hays, *The Faith of Jesus Christ*, p. 293.
[68] Hays, *The Faith of Jesus Christ*, p. 293.
[69] Hays, *The Faith of Jesus Christ*, p. 293.
[70] Hays, *The Faith of Jesus Christ*, p. 294.
[71] Hays, *The Faith of Jesus Christ*, p. 294.

view, this has the distinct advantage of explaining how Pauline ethics is christologically grounded . . ." while "from a practical point of view, this has the distinct advantage of summoning us to live lives of costly sacrificial burden-bearing."[72]

Putting these concerns together, we might summarize them as the simultaneous rejection of a set of opposed errors. On one hand, protest is being raised against a kind of quasi-Pelagian theological anthropology and soteriology that might offer a Christology that reduces to (or, minimally, emphasizes and highlights) an exemplarist view of atonement. Hays is stoutly opposed to any interpretation that would deny or even downplay the historical significance and indeed the ultimacy of what Christ did on behalf of others. Thus he worries that the traditional anthropological interpretation mistakenly puts the emphasis either on the actions (or "works") of individual followers of Jesus or on the dispositional attitudes of these followers. Hays's opposition is clear: "by no means should this be understood to mean that Christians are saved by their own Herculean faithfulness"; to the contrary, "the central emphasis of the christological interpretation of πίστις' Ιαου Χριστου is precisely that we are saved by Jesus' faithfulness, not by our own cognitive disposition or confessional orthodoxy."[73] He worries that the anthropological interpretation places the emphasis on the "salvific efficacy of individual faith or even to turn faith into a bizarre sort of work, in which Christians jump through the entranceway of salvation by cultivating the right sort of spiritual disposition," and instead he insists that salvation is "won" by the faithfulness of Christ on behalf of others.[74] Thus, "because justification hinges upon this action of Jesus Christ, upon an event *extra nos*, it is a terrible and ironic blunder to read Paul as though his gospel made redemption contingent upon our act of deciding to dispose ourselves toward God in a particular way."[75]

On the other hand, Hays is also opposed to any view of salvation that would undercut the pressing and urgent need for a Christologically focused ethics or that would even allow for complacency. If I understand him correctly, Hays is exercised to oppose any notions that would say, in effect, "well, Jesus did it all for us, so clearly there is nothing else left to do that matters for salvation" or "since the faith and faithfulness of Jesus are what

---

[72] Hays, *The Faith of Jesus Christ*, p. 294, citing Sam Williams, "Again *Pistis Christou*," *Catholic Biblical Quarterly* 49 (1987), p. 444.

[73] Hays, *The Faith of Jesus Christ*, p. 293.   [74] Hays, *The Faith of Jesus Christ*, p. 293.

[75] Hays, *The Faith of Jesus Christ*, p. 211.

really matters, then while it would of course be good if my faith and faithfulness were to mirror or otherwise resemble his, to suppose that this has anything to do with my salvation is to undervalue what he believed and did for me." To summarize, on one hand Hays is concerned to resist any soteriologies that would see Christ's faith and faithfulness as important in an exemplary sense but that would elevate human agency (in belief and obedience) and thus make that human agency ultimate in salvation. But on the other hand, Hays also opposes those soteriologies that would undercut the need for genuine faith and faithful obedience.

What are we to make of these concerns? Hays is pessimistic about the resources of traditional (especially Protestant) theology on this point, but he is also cautious about the explanatory scope and power of his own proposal. Is Hays right that the objective genitive or anthropological interpretation leads to theological problems? Is he warranted in holding out hope that his own preferred subjective genitive or Christological reading will avoid such problems?

2.5.2 Reaching Backward and Moving Forward: *Ressourcement* and Theological Interpretation

It is not immediately clear that the objective genitive approach entails such theological problems. Perhaps it opens the door to such problems; maybe it allows for them if other theological safeguards are not in place. But any relationships of necessity or inevitability are less than pellucid. Nor is it immediately obvious that the subjective genitive interpretation always avoids the problems. To the contrary, it seems that the Christological account may allow for—or perhaps even promote—the loss of concern for human responsibility and the ethical imperatives that characterize Pauline (and, more broadly, New Testament) theology: if one is saved by the faithfulness of Christ whether or not one has faith or exhibits covenantal fidelity in obedience, then such faith and fidelity are clearly not necessary for salvation.

But what if a response of human faith and faithful obedience is necessary *in some sense*—but perhaps is not necessary in *another sense*? It seems to me that Hays is making the right affirmations—I am with him on these points and think that Christians today should resist the errors that he critiques. But some further work needs to be done, and in this instance I propose to do what the medieval scholastics did: when facing a dilemma, draw a distinction.

Analytic theology might help in doing so—and, indeed, the analytic theology of an earlier generation did just this sort of hard and careful work. To access this earlier work, I shall draw upon some of the relevant seventeenth-century distinctions and developments in the debates about faith and good works in salvation. With these tools, I propose a way forward—one that seeks to satisfy the important soteriological desiderata that Hays so helpfully articulates.

First, the traditional distinction between justification and salvation is both warranted and important. Justification really is distinct from salvation; on various versions of the New Perspective on Paul and on traditional doctrines as well, justification is an important element of the doctrine of salvation, but it is not the whole of it. I take it that there is nothing very controversial about this; I am only clarifying what I take to be deeply rooted in Christian tradition and fairly obvious on even very brief reflection.

Second, πίστις Χριστου is the cause of justification. But immediately we must distinguish and clarify. Initially, we must clarify what we mean by *cause*. Here is where the distinctions of older scholastic theology are helpful: when we say that Christ is the cause of the justification of sinners, we mean that he is the *meritorious* cause. Indeed, Christ is the *sole meritorious* cause, and "salvation is a freely given gift that rests on God's grace alone in Christ."[76] Neither human behavior ("works") or human cognitive states ("belief") can be said to be all or part of such a cause.

Beyond this, we must also be clear about what we mean by πίστις Χριστου at this point. Earlier I noted that πίστις Χριστου could be construed as:

(α) human belief and trust in Jesus Christ;
(β) trusting and faithful human obedience to Jesus Christ;
(γ) the trusting belief of Jesus Christ;
(δ) the trusting and faithful obedience of Jesus Christ.

What do I mean when I say that πίστις Χριστου is meritorious for salvation? I am talking about (δ). The trusting and faithful obedience of the incarnate Son makes justification possible and actual. Note that we need not, at this point, make a decision about (γ) one way or the other; whether or not Christ enjoys the beatific vision, it is his faithful obedience—what the

---

[76] Richard A. Muller, *Dictionary of Latin and Greek Theological Terms, Drawn Principally from Protestant Scholastic Theology* (Grand Rapids: Baker Academic, 1985), p. 63.

Protestant scholastics sometimes referred to as the *active* and *passive* right-eousness of Christ—that brings about the justification of the sinner.

Does this mean that the "subjective" or Christological reading is correct? Are we then to conclude that (α) and (β) are inert with respect to justification? Do they play no causal role? Is what humans *believe*—and indeed what they *do* and how they *live*—thus somehow irrelevant to justification (and perhaps, more broadly, to salvation)? Surely our affirmation of (δ) as the meritorious cause of justification would address and assuage Hays's concern to insist that "we are saved by Jesus' faithfulness." But does this affirmation not make our position vulnerable to Hays's other big concern?

This brings us to our next affirmation: human faith is *also* rightly under-stood as a cause of justification: (α) is an *instrumental cause*. To be clear, it is not a meritorious cause; on the contrary, it is only an instrumental cause. But it is a cause nonetheless. Thus we should think of (α), at least in normal or default cases, as divinely ordained and indeed as necessary for justification.

But have we yet adequately addressed Hays's second major concern? It is not clear that we have yet done so, for to affirm only (α) and (δ) still leaves us with Hays's important concern to account for the reality and necessity of a genuine Christian—and thus *Christocentric*—ethic. If what counts is only what Christ did, then does what I *do* really matter? Indeed, if what Jesus did and believed is all that really matters, then does what I *believe* really matter? The clear and unwavering answer should be: Yes, indeed; yes it does. How we live when joined in union with Christ indeed does matter, and not only for Christian witness or Christian assurance. So we need to say more: πίστις Χριστου is also necessary for salvation when considered more broadly, and here we should think of such faith as nothing short of (β). Faithful obedience really is necessary for salvation, for "the obedience of faith" is part of salvation (Rom 1:5).

It might at this point help to recall traditional Reformed (and, for that matter, Lutheran) doctrines of good works.[77] For the Reformed also insist that good works are necessary for salvation. Human good works do not justify sinners, but they are vitally important and indeed necessary for salvation. This much is plain in early modern Reformed theology: Francis Turretin speaks for the broad Reformed tradition when he answers the question "Are good works necessary for salvation?" with an unambiguous

---

[77] See further the discussion in Thomas H. McCall and Keith D. Stanglin, *After Arminius: A Historical Introduction to Arminian Theology* (New York: Oxford University Press, forth-coming).

"We affirm."[78] A core affirmation is that such good works are necessary as the evidence or "fruit" of salvation. As Amandus Polanus puts it, good works are the necessary demonstration of living and vital faith.[79]

Beyond such basic but important agreement, however, various Reformed scholastics take different positions on just *how* good works are necessary. In addition to being the *evidence* of salvation, some take good works to be the *means* of salvation, others add that it is a *condition* of salvation, and some will go so far as to say that good works are a *cause* of salvation.

Among some Reformed theologians (both Anglican and continental), there is a further distinction drawn between the necessity of cause and the necessity of means. It is a commonplace to insist that good works are necessary as the *means* of receiving salvation. Thus John Edwards maintains that good works are necessary to salvation, and Henry Compton says that "it is agreed by all sober men, that a virtuous and holy life is necessary to salvation, not as giving a right, but as the necessary means to obtain that right, which is purchased by Christ's blood."[80] Major continental Reformed theologians are in agreement; Johannes Wollebius, for instance, also insists that the principal efficient cause of good works is the Holy Spirit and that their instrumental cause is faith.[81] Importantly, while Wollebius denies that good works are necessary with respect to soteriological merit, he does insist that such good works are, strictly speaking, necessary with respect to *precept* and *means*.[82] As someone who comes into an inheritance must travel to the city where it is located in order to receive it, so also a sinner must perform good works to obtain salvation—not as anything meritorious or that makes one deserving of that inheritance, but as a necessary *means* to the reception of it.[83] Edward Reynolds takes the same view. But his deployment of a very similar analogy actually makes it seem as

---

[78] Francis Turretin, *Institutio Theologiae Elencticae, Pars Secunda* XVII.III (Geneva, 1582), p. 768; Francis Turretin, *Institutes of Elenctic Theology* Vol. 2, translated by George Musgrave Giger, edited by James T. Dennison, Jr. (Philipsburg: P&R Publishing, 1994), p. 702.

[79] Amandus Polanus, *Collegium Anti-Bellarminianum* (Basel, 1613), p. 101. *Evangelici falso accusantur a Bellarmino quali neget bonoru operum necessitate. Nam etsi neget bona opera esse causa salutis, non negant tamen eadem esse necessaria ad demonstrandam vivan fidem, per quam servamur.*

[80] Cited in Stephen Hampton, *Anti-Arminians: The Anglican Reformed Tradition from Charles II to George I* (Oxford: Oxford University Press, 2008), p. 124.

[81] Johannes Wollebius, *Christianae theologiae compendium* II.I.iii (Amsterdam, 1655), p. 291.

[82] Wollebius, *Christianae theologiae compendium* II.I.xv, p. 295. *Necessaria sunt bona opera, necessitate praecepti et medii, non autem necessitate causae et meriti.*

[83] Wollebius, *Christianae theologiae compendium* II.xv., p. 295. Cf. Samuel Rutherford, *A Survey of the Spirituall Antichrist* (London, 1648), pp. 62–63.

though works are a *precondition*: a customer who buys property must actually travel to that property in order to acquire it.[84]

This means that many of the Reformed make works a *condition*—indeed, a condition *sine qua non*—for salvation more generally. Hampton notes that Edwards even goes so far as to say that Paul "separates works from justification, yet he doth not separate them from justifying faith."[85] Petrus van Mastricht says that good works are necessary not only by divine command but also as conditions.[86] Stephen Hampton notes that the Reformed Anglican theologian "[Thomas] Barlow requires from the believer exactly what [George] Bull required, but he requires it for salvation, not for justification."[87]

Some Reformed theologians do not shrink from referring to good works as a *cause* of salvation. Hieronymous Zanchi holds that good works are an instrumental cause.[88] Samuel Rutherford agrees; good works have a causal instrumental power.[89] Gisjbert Voetius says that it is better to understand good works as instrumentally causal rather than efficiently causal, but they indeed are rightly said to play a causal role.[90] Beyond this, Johannes Piscator will even go so far as to say that such good works have the nature of an efficient (though inferior) cause.[91] As one who is given a treasure buried on a mountain must not only climb the mountain but also dig the treasure in order to receive this gift, so also the one who receives the free gift of salvation must perform good works.[92]

Heinrich Alsted says that good works are necessary not only by divine mandate but also as a medium or means in the way of salvation (*via*

---

[84] See the discussion in Hampton, *Anti-Arminians*, pp. 124–125.

[85] John Edwards, *Discourse of Faith and Justification*, p. 197, as noted in Hampton, *Anti-Arminians*, p. 123.

[86] Petrus van Mastricht, *Theoretico-Practiica Theologia, editio secunda* VI.VIII.XXVII (Utrecht: 1698), pp. 744–745. See the discussion in Hampton, *Anti-Arminians*, pp. 88, 115. See further the discussion by Ryan M. Hurd, "*Dei Via Regia*: The Westminster Divine Anthony Tuckney on the Necessity of Works for Salvation," *Westminster Theological Journal* (2019), pp. 1–17.

[87] Hampton, *Anti-Arminians*, p. 99.

[88] Hieronymous Zanchi, *De Natura Dei, Seu De Divinis Attributis* V.2.III (Nuestadt: 1593), p. 670.

[89] Samuel Rutherford, *Examen Arminianismi* (Utrecht: 1668), pp. 532–533.

[90] Gisbert Voetius, *Thersites Heautontimorenos hoc est Remonstrantum Hyperaspistes* (Utrecht: 1635), p. 168.

[91] Johannes Piscator, *Analysis Logica Sex Epistolarum Pauli, editio secunda* (n.p., 1593), p. 88.

[92] Johannes Piscator, cited in William Forbes, *Considerationes Modestae et Pacificae Contoversiarum* (Oxford: 1850), pp. 312–313.

salutis)—and even as a necessary condition and cause (*conditio & causa sine qua non*).[93] Turretin's summary is apt:

> Works can be considered three ways: either with reference to justification or sanctification or glorification. They are related to justification not antecedently, efficiently, and meritoriously, but consequently and declaratively. They are related to sanctification constitutively because they constitute and promote it. They are related to glorification antecedently and ordinatively because they are related to it as the means to the end ... [94]

But, wait, does not all this talk about "conditions" involve commitment to a "contractual" approach that is reviled as the root of so much theological evil? Does this not somehow entail the conclusion that human sinners must somehow first act so as to earn grace? Does not the affirmation of "conditions"—in just any sense—entail the conclusion that God must be "conditioned" into adopting a posture of mercy toward humans? In a word, the answer is *No*. The grace of God is rightly and properly understood to be, in John M. G. Barclay's way of putting it, *unconditioned*.[95] God's grace is fundamentally prior and is always ultimate. Indeed, one can follow my suggestions and (to employ Barclay's categories) hold that God's grace is marked by superabundance, singularity, priority, incongruity, efficacy, and even—understood in the proper sense—non-circularity.[96] Grace is superabundant; where sin increased, grace increased all the more (Rom 5:20–21). Grace is singular in the sense that it is motivated by the sheer and simple goodness of God.[97] There is a fundamental priority of grace in salvation, for it enables a genuine human response. Grace is incongruous in the sense that it is offered "without regard for the worth of the recipient."[98] Grace is efficacious in the sense that it does for the recipient what the recipient cannot do for herself. And grace can even be said to be non-circular in the sense that it does not establish any sort of *quid pro quo;* God does not give in order that God might receive something needed by God. But a proper relationship with God—a relationship of the kind shared between

---

[93] Johannes-Heinrich Alsted, *Theologica Polemica* (Hanover, 1620), p. 496.

[94] Turretin, *Institutes of Elenctic Theology*, Vol. 2, p. 705.

[95] John M. G. Barclay, *Paul and the Gift* (Grand Rapids: William B. Eerdmans Publishing Co., 2015).

[96] Barclay, *Paul and the Gift*, pp. 70–75.

[97] I do not mean that grace is "singular" in the sense that "it is incompatible with notions of divine judgment and wrath," cf. Barclay, *Paul and the Gift*, p. 140.

[98] Barclay, *Paul and the Gift*, p. 73.

persons—may yet have conditions and thus be *conditional* even if the grace that seeks and enables that relationship is *unconditioned*. Indeed, even those who reject "conditionality"—no matter how forcefully—are not always entirely consistent.[99] For instance, Chris Tilling says of Douglas Campbell's view that "the big issue for Campbell is that faith *not* be understood...as the *condition* for salvation."[100] Campbell himself, however, also says that faith "is necessary if final life or salvation is to be reached."[101] But if faith is a *necessary condition*, then surely it is a *condition*.

Still, some may argue that this way of addressing Hays's second major desideratum makes us once again vulnerable to the first. The worry might be that we are somehow thrown back upon ourselves to make this happen. Is this a legitimate concern? It might be—depending upon what other theological resources are available. But for the Trinitarian theologian—the theologian who has a robust account of the necessity and efficacy of the work of the Holy Spirit—the short and decisive answer is No! In no sense are human sinners left to somehow repair or save themselves—or even to start the process of salvation. For the Holy Spirit is the active agent who graciously enables the response of faith and faithfulness. Thomas F. Torrance explains the formulation given by Basil of Caesarea:

> However, Basil drew a distinction between the work of the Father as "the original cause" (τὴν προκαταρκτικὴν αἰτίαν) of all created things, and the work of the Son as "the operative cause" (τὴν δημιουργικὴν αἰτίαν), and the work of the Holy Spirit as "the perfecting cause" (τὴν τελειωτιὴν αἰτίαν)...Thus in upholding living, rational creatures from below and within them and in bringing them to their true end or telos in God the Holy Spirit makes them participate in the very life and holiness of God himself.[102]

---

[99] Barclay's work is both well-informed and theologically fecund, and it awaits further theological analysis. For an interesting conversation that probes some of these matters further, see Ben Witherington III, *Biblical Theology: The Convergence of the Canon* (Cambridge: Cambridge University Press, 2019), pp. 395–401.

[100] Chris Tilling, "Campbell's Faith: Advancing the *Pistis Christou* Debate," in Chris Tilling, ed., *Beyond Old and New Perspectives on Paul: Reflections on the Work of Douglas Campbell* (Eugene: Cascade, 2014), p. 237.

[101] Campbell, *The Deliverance of God*, p. 68.

[102] Thomas F. Torrance, *The Trinitarian Faith: The Evangelical Theology of the Ancient Catholic Church* (Edinburgh: T&T Clark, 1988), pp. 228–229.

The Holy Spirit enables the faith-filled and faithful response of redeemed and justified sinners, the Holy Spirit cooperates with the responsive human agent throughout to bring the person into conformity with Christ, and the Holy Spirit brings the human person to perfection in grace.

2.6 Conclusion

So where does this leave us with respect to the πίστις Χριστου debate? It leaves us in position to affirm the main lines of Hooker's interpretation—as this reading is augmented with analytic theological resources drawn from the tradition of Protestant scholasticism. Recall that Hooker makes the following points. First, the "phrase could convey both meanings simultaneously."[103] Second, the debate must be resolved at a theological (rather than merely exegetical) level. Third, while both the subjective and objective dimensions are included, it should be clear that the Christological element is (logically) prior and paramount: that "faith/faithfulness is primarily that of Christ, and we share in it only because we are in him."[104] And, fourth, this faith "works"; it produces actions of faithful allegiance and obedience: "in Christ, and through him, we are able to share his trust and obedience, and so become what God called his people to be."[105] I think that Hooker is correct on all these points, and theological resources retrieved from the tradition help fill out the proposal. With these resources, finally, we arrive at an account that is both consistent with the relevant exegetical considerations and that can satisfy the important theological desiderata.

---

[103] Hooker, "Another Look," p. 48.   [104] Hooker, "Another Look," p. 62.
[105] Hooker, "Another Look," p. 62.

3

The Identity of the Son

The Incarnation and the Freedom of God

3.1 Introduction

"Recently the world of Barth studies has been rocked by an internal debate." With these words, George Hunsinger begins a book that continues and sharpens this very debate.[1] My interests are not in this debate as such; my primary concerns are not with the question of the proper interpretation of Karl Barth. I am, of course, interested in what Barth had to say about these matters (as he was a very important modern theologian), and naturally I would rather have the right interpretation rather than a mistaken one. But I am much more interested in the theological issues raised by this debate, and accordingly I shall use the current "Barth wars" as an entry-point into the issues. In other words, my goal here is not to persuade anyone that I have the right reading of Barth; instead it is to explore the fascinating and important theological issues that have surfaced in this debate.

To this end, in this chapter I shall first introduce the debate; here I shall offer a descriptive overview of the debate as it has developed and spread. Following this I shall offer a theological analysis of the "revisionist" reading of Barth's work, and to this end I shall probe the exegetical basis for the view by asking what theological interpretation of Scripture contributes to the debate, I shall explore issues of coherence, and I shall raise some serious theological concerns that accompany the revisionist proposal.

3.2 McCormack's Gambit

A seminal essay by Bruce L. McCormack on the proper understanding of Karl Barth's view of election ignited the current debate. Eventually some key

[1] George Hunsinger, *Reading Barth with Charity: A Hermeneutical Proposal* (Grand Rapids: Baker Academic, 2015), p. xi.

Analytic Christology and the Theological Interpretation of the New Testament. Thomas H. McCall, Oxford University Press (2021). © Thomas H. McCall. DOI: 10.1093/oso/9780198857495.003.0004

issues and questions were clarified, and it became clearer where the revisionist proposal was simply and directly an interpretation of Barth and where McCormack's own views were pressing further in the direction given by (the mature) Barth. Perhaps a brief survey of these developments will be helpful.

3.2.1 The Barth Wars: The Opening Salvo

In his essay "Grace and Being," McCormack makes a series of arresting claims.[2] He begins with the assertion that "when the history of theology in the twentieth century is written from the vantage point of, say, one hundred years from now, I am confident that the greatest contribution of Karl Barth to the development of church doctrine will be located in his doctrine of election."[3] This is because, as McCormack sees things, Barth's doctrine of election has such profound consequences not only for an understanding of predestination and salvation but also—and much more importantly—for the doctrine of God. Barth gives us nothing short of a "revolution," and this revolution is "a revolution in the doctrine of God."[4] The biggest impact of Barth's account is not, then, in soteriology but in theological "ontology."

Barth offers a stark alternative to historic Reformed doctrines of predestination and election. Famously, Barth insists that Jesus Christ is both the Object and the Subject of election. While the older accounts were able to conceive of Christ as the Mediator between God and humanity and thus could possibly be rendered consistent with Barth's insistence that Christ is the Subject of election, these older accounts had no place for his recognition of Jesus Christ as the Object of election. As McCormack points out, Barth had deep concerns about the scholastic Reformed teaching. At one level, the classic Reformed teaching that posits a strictly limited account of election (according to which God eternally decrees that a specific number of particular persons will be saved while the others are not saved by God) was rejected by Barth, and in its place he offered a universal account of election. But, as McCormack notes, the question of "who gets in?" is a "secondary question" for Barth, for "what is primary" is the question "who is this God

---

[2] Bruce L. McCormack, "Grace and Being: The Role of God's Gracious Election in Karl Barth's Theological Ontology," in John Webster, ed., *The Cambridge Companion to Karl Barth* (Cambridge: Cambridge University Press, 2000), pp. 92–110.
[3] McCormack, "Grace and Being," p. 92.   [4] McCormack, "Grace and Being," p. 93.

who elects and what does a knowledge of this God tell us about the nature of election?"[5] In place of the standard Reformed account, Barth offers a distinctly *Christological* account of the doctrine. On McCormack's reading, Barth rejects abstract and speculative notions of the pre-existent second person of the Trinity as the *logos asarkos*; if Barth is to allow any talk at all of a *logos asarkos*, it will be only as we think of the Son as *logos incarnandus* (the Word to-be-incarnated) and further only as the identity of that Son is constituted by his humanity as God-for-us.[6] He says that Barth's doctrine of election, with its "eternal act of establishing a covenant of grace," has real "ontological significance."[7] It has this significance because God's act of decision to be God-for-us and God-with-us is "an act of Self-determination."[8] Barth's distinctly Christological doctrine of election thus comes into direct conflict with Calvin's doctrine, and the divide goes much deeper than the extent of election (and the possibility of reprobation of sinful humans). Because the divine act of election establishes God as the God who is for and with humanity—even to the extent of Jesus Christ being God-forsaken—on Barth's view, the difference goes all the way to theological ontology. For Calvin, and the Reformed scholastics more generally, are trapped by an "essentialist" ontology, while Barth's Christological doctrine leads him to embrace an "actualist" ontology.[9] What does this mean for our understanding of the nature of God? "In what sense, then, is the incarnation of the 'Son' and the outpouring of the Holy Spirit 'constitutive' of the eternal being of God?"[10] After working to distinguish this view from that of Hegel, McCormack answers that the decision of election—the decision to be God-for-us and God-with-us—is constitutive of God's being "in this sense only: as a consequence of the primal decision in which God assigned to himself the being that he would have throughout eternity (a being-for the human race), God is already in pre-temporal eternity – *by way of anticipation* – that which he would become in time."[11] In his own summary: "to say that 'Jesus Christ' is the Subject of election is to say that there is no *Logos asarkos* in the absolute sense of a mode of existence in the second 'person' of the Trinity which is independent of the determination for incarnation; no 'eternal Son'

---

[5] McCormack, "Grace and Being," p. 93.
[6] McCormack, "Grace and Being," pp. 93–95.
[7] McCormack, "Grace and Being," p. 98.   [8] McCormack, "Grace and Being," p. 98.
[9] McCormack, "Grace and Being," p. 98. On "actualism," see also George Hunsinger, *How To Read Karl Barth: The Shape of His Theology* (Oxford: Oxford University Press, 1991), pp. 30–32.
[10] McCormack, "Grace and Being," p. 100.
[11] McCormack, "Grace and Being," p. 100.

if that Son is seen in abstraction from the gracious election in which God determined and determines never to be a God apart from the human race. The second 'person' of the Trinity has a name and His name is Jesus Christ."[12]

McCormack then explores the implications of Barth's view of election for his doctrine of the Trinity. He inquires as to the "logical relation of God's gracious election to the triunity of God."[13] He observes that Barth never addresses this question directly, and he admits that Barth's statements are not entirely consistent with respect to this issue. Nor can the inconsistencies simply be explained (away) as development of doctrine or change of mind, for competing claims are made even deep in Barth's corpus. As McCormack says, "the only conclusion I have been able to come to is that Barth either did not fully realize the profound implications of his doctrine of election for the doctrine of the Trinity, or he shied away from drawing them for reasons known only to himself."[14] But where Barth may have been hesitant to do so, McCormack is not. Instead, he offers a "critical correction" of Barth:

> The denial of the existence of a *Logos asarkos* in any other sense than the concrete one of a being of the Logos as *incarnandus*, the affirmation that Jesus Christ is the second 'person' of the Trinity and the concomitant rejection of any free-floating talk of the 'eternal Son' as a mythological abstraction – these commitments require that we see the triunity of God logically as a function of divine election. Expressed more exactly: the eternal act of Self-differentiation in which God is God 'a second time in a very different way' (CD I/1, pp. 316, 324) and a third time as well, is *given in* the eternal act in which God elects himself for the human race. The *decision* for the covenant of grace is the ground of God's triunity and, therefore, of the eternal generation of the Son and of the eternal procession of the Holy Spirit from Father and Son. In other words, the works of God *ad intra* (the trinitarian processions) find their ground in the *first* of the works of God *ad extra* (viz. election).[15]

Thus God's triunity is logically consequent to, and dependent upon, God's decision to be God-for-and-with-us. Surely McCormack is correct about this one point at least: compared with patristic, medieval, and Reformation theologies, this truly is a "revolutionary" doctrine.

---

[12] McCormack, "Grace and Being," p. 100.
[14] McCormack, "Grace and Being," p. 102.
[13] McCormack, "Grace and Being," p. 101.
[15] McCormack, "Grace and Being," p. 103.

3.2.2 The Empire Strikes Back: Responses to the "Revisionist" Proposal

The reactions to McCormack's proposal have been mixed, but they have not been tepid. Several theologians (some working as interpreters of Barth and others as constructive theologians) have been supportive of his proposal either in whole or in part.[16] But several critics have emerged, and some of them have reacted quite forcefully.

Many of the criticisms are centered on the proper interpretation of Barth. George Hunsinger and Paul D. Molnar (among others) have been particularly exercised to show that McCormack's revisionist interpretation of Barth is mistaken. They work to show that not only does Barth never draw the "implications" and conclusions drawn by McCormack—Barth also, repeatedly and forcefully, continues to resist and even explicitly *deny* the positions held by McCormack. The conclusion to one of Hunsinger's important essays is representative of such counter-arguments (with respect to tone as well as content):

> Nor did Barth change his mind on this score over the course of writing his *Church Dogmaics* – another dubious claim that, although easy to assert, has not been proven. The notion that the eternal Son was constituted by pre-temporal election was something so bizarre – and obviously false – that Barth could see little point in pausing very long to refute it. He did, however, make at least this statement: "Daß Jesus Christus der Sohn Gottes ist, daß beruht freilich nicht auf Erwählung" (*KD* II/2, 114) ["Of course, the fact that Jesus Christ *is* the Son of God does not rest on election" (*CD* II/2, 107 rev.)]. Barth's "of course" (*freilich*) should have been sufficient in itself to make the argument of this essay unnecessary.[17]

---

[16] E.g., Paul Dafydd Jones, "Obedience, Trinity, and Election: Thinking With and Beyond the *Church Dogmatics*," in Michael T. Dempsey, ed., *Trinity and Election in Contemporary Theology* (Grand Rapids: William B. Eerdmans Publishing Co., 2011), pp. 138–161; *The Humanity of Christ: Christology in Karl Barth's Church Dogmatics* (London: Continuum/T&T Clark, 2008); Paul T. Nimmo, "Barth and the Election-Trinity Debate: A Pneumatological View," in Michael T. Dempsey, ed., *Trinity and Election in Contemporary Theology* (Grand Rapids: William B. Eerdmans Publishing Co., 2011), pp. 162–181; Aaron T. Smith, "God's Self-Specification: His Being Is His Electing," in Michael T. Dempsey, ed., *Trinity and Election in Contemporary Theology* (Grand Rapids: William B. Eerdmans Publishing Co., 2011), pp. 201–225.

[17] George Hunsinger, "Election and the Trinity: Twenty-Five Theses on the Theology of Karl Barth," in Michael T. Dempsey, ed., *Trinity and Election in Contemporary Theology* (Grand Rapids: William B. Eerdmans Publishing Co., 2011), p. 114. See also especially Paul D. Molnar,

Moreover, not only do McCormack and the other revisionists misread Barth, Hunsinger alleges that they do so in a way that is fundamentally uncharitable, for they read him as self-contradictory and indeed incoherent.[18]

Moving beyond the complaints about the revisionist tendency to misinterpret Barth, however, there are more substantive theological concerns. Some critics worry that McCormack's proposal opens the door to the very possibility that he so clearly wants to rule out: this is the God who is "behind the back of Jesus."[19] McCormack is exercised to follow Barth's insistence that God is truly revealed in Jesus Christ, thus there is nothing to God's being—no inscrutable *Decretum Absolutum*—that is in any way contrary to or even different from the God revealed in the person of Christ. And yet the worry arises that McCormack's own proposal somehow allows and invites the very speculation that the theory is meant to overcome. For if God *elects* his triunity, then there must be something prior to this Trinity that chooses to be God in this way. And, if so, then we have, in Molnar's words, "the specter of an unknown God behind the being of the eternal Trinity."[20] Several critics are concerned that McCormack's proposal basically reduces to a version of Hegelianism. McCormack is alert to this concern, and has been from the beginning of the debates; he denies that his starting place or motivation is that of Hegel's, he argues that significant elements of Barth's (and his) view differ sharply from those of Hegel, and he also points out that Barth was, by his own admission, not entirely allergic to Hegel but able to adapt what was good and even fond of doing "a little Hegeling."[21] But the critics are not satisfied; Edwin Chr. van Driel is concerned that even if the motivations differ and there are some differences, nonetheless it is hard to "see how McCormack would end up at a different place than Hegel, even if his starting place – will rather than nature – is different."[22]

Faith, Freedom and the Spirit: The Economic Trinity in Barth, Torrance, and Contemporary Theology (Downers Grove: InterVarsity Academic, 2015), pp. 129–312.

[18] E.g., George Hunsinger, *Reading Barth with Charity: A Hermenuetical Proposal* (Grand Rapids: Baker Academic, 2015), pp. xii–xiii.

[19] The phrase ("behind the back of Jesus") is from Thomas Torrance, but the basic concern is one that resonates deeply with McCormack as well. See Thomas F. Torrance, *The Christian Doctrine of God: One Being, Three Persons* (Edinburgh: T&T Clark, 1996), p. 5.

[20] Molnar, *Faith, Freedom and the Spirit*, p. 174.

[21] E.g., McCormack, "Grace and Being," pp. 99–100; Bruce L. McCormack, *Orthodox and Modern: Studies in the Theology of Karl Barth* (Grand Rapids: Baker Academic, 2008), p. 271.

[22] Edwin Chr. van Driel, "Karl Barth on the Eternal Existence of Jesus Christ," *Scottish Journal of Theology* 60:1 (2007), p. 54. See also Molnar, *Faith, Freedom and the Spirit*, p. 258.

Other criticisms are more serious. Molnar charges McCormack of trans-gressing the boundaries of creedal Christology: he "avoids the clutches of Apollinarianism only to fall into the open arms of Nestorian thinking (that could at any moment become monophysite)."[23] And, as if this is not enough, there is more—Molnar charges the revisionist account with Arianism too; he refers to Kevin Hector's engagement as amounting to "the perfect assertion of Arian subordinationism" and concludes that on this account the Son's "*homoousion* with the Father has been negated."[24]

In my view, van Driel raises some of the most interesting and important concerns. He asks several probing questions. "First, if divine election is an essential act of the divine will, constitutive of the divine being, how can McCormack avoid the idea that *creation* is likewise essential to God and constitutive of the divine being?"[25] After all, he reasons, if incarnation is essential to God and constitutes the divine being, then—since incarnation presupposes a *carnis* and thus a creation of *carnis*—then it follows that creation is essential to God. His second concern is this: "If election and incarnation logically and ontologically precede the triune nature and God's attributes, then what, on McCormack's proposal, makes it possible for God to elect and to give God to what is not God?"[26] If a decision to be the-Triune-God-for-and-with-us-as-incarnate precedes the reality not only of the incarnation but also the Trinity, then *something or someone* is doing the deciding. Moreover, it must have some set of properties or attributes to be able to do so; minimally, it must have the capacity and power to choose, to be a decider. He notes that "this leads to a third problem: not only what properties, but what subject precedes the divine choice?"[27] It is difficult to see how the possibility of self-constitution can be sustained on this account, thus it is threatened by self-referential incoherence.

I shall not pursue at any length the issues related to the proper interpret-ation of Barth. I pass by these for several reasons. First, and most fundamen-tally, I am interested in the substantive theological issues at stake, and I think that we do well to avoid the temptation to think that the *telos* of theological investigation is the proper interpretation of Barth (or any other theologians

---

[23] Molnar, *Faith, Freedom and the Spirit*, p. 253. If Molnar is correct, then McCormack has notched a rather remarkable achievement by simultaneously embracing a heresy and coming close to embracing the opposite heresy.

[24] Molnar, *Faith, Freedom and the Spirit*, pp. 170–171.

[25] van Driel, "Karl Barth on the Eternal Existence of Jesus Christ," p. 54.

[26] van Driel, "Karl Barth on the Eternal Existence of Jesus Christ," p. 54.

[27] van Driel, "Karl Barth on the Eternal Existence of Jesus Christ," p. 54.

of the tradition, no matter how much they are deserving of respect). Second, I think that it is quite possible that there is some ambiguity and possibly even some inconsistency within Barth's own corpus (and even with the *Dogmatics*) on this point. As van Driel notes, "the problem lies, not so much in McCormack's reading, but in an ambiguity in the formulations of Barth himself."[28] It may simply be the case that McCormack and his fellow revisionists are straightening out Barth in a more Hegel-friendly (I do not say "Hegelian," for there are important differences) way while Hunsinger, Molnar and others are straightening out Barth in a more classical way.[29] Third, McCormack is well aware that he is taking leave of Barth at various points. He knows that Barth (even the mature Barth, even after Vol. II) did not draw the revisionist conclusions. He has recognized this point from the beginning, and he readily admits that he is going "beyond" Barth even as he goes "with" him.[30] He says very clearly that his "own work has used Barth as a resource (the *primary* resource)" for his own constructive work. He does so with good reason: in his view, "Karl Barth was the greatest theologian since the Reformation. But we do him no service if we simply repeat him. For his interest lay in the subject matter to which he bore witness..."[31] Thus it seems to me that some of the criticisms about his interpretation of Barth are less than fair and allow the various parties to talk past one another. And, at any rate, the important theological issues are much more interesting.

3.2.3 McCormack's Constructive Proposal

In some cases, the debates to this point seem to have generated as much heat as light. But if anything good has come from these debates, perhaps it is this:

---

[28] van Driel, "Karl Barth on the Eternal Existence of Jesus Christ," p. 56. Cf. Paul Dafydd Jones, "Obedience, Trinity, and Election: Thinking With and Beyond the *Church Dogmatics*," in Michael T. Dempsey, ed., *Trinity and Election in Contemporary Theology* (Grand Rapids: William B. Eerdmans Publishing Co., 2011), pp. 138–161. Jones admits that Barth's work is "patient of multiple interpretations," and while he identifies as a "revisionist," he is "obliged to admit the viability of 'traditionalist' readings," p. 157.

[29] Alternatively, Brandon Gallaher maintains that we should leave the tension in Barth unresolved out of respect for him as a truly "dialectical" theologian. See Brandon Gallaher, *Freedom and Necessity in Modern Trinitarian Theology* (Oxford: Oxford University Press, 2016), pp. 122–141.

[30] E.g., Bruce L. McCormack, "Election and the Trinity: Theses in Response to George Hunsinger," in Michael T. Dempsey, *Trinity and Election in Contemporary Theology* (Grand Rapids: William B. Eerdmans Publishing Co., 2011), pp. 134–137.

[31] McCormack, "Theses in Response to George Hunsinger," p. 137.

the revisionists have been encouraged and enabled to clarify and (in some cases, at least) qualify the proposal. We can see clearly enough that McCormack and the revisionists simultaneously claim support for their proposal in the theology of Barth and admit that they are going beyond him on the basis of his profound insights. We can also see with more clarity where the revisionist account contrasts with more traditional theology (and here I mean "traditional" not merely in the sense of older readings of Barth but the deep Christian tradition). Where the traditional account holds that God's existence as Triune is necessary, the revisionist proposal does not find this to be so straightforward. Where traditional doctrine sees the Trinity as necessary and creation and incarnation as contingent, the revisionist view sees them as going together. Where traditional theology is confident that the Trinity (logically and chronologically) precedes election, on McCormack's view the doctrine of election precedes the doctrine of the Trinity. On the traditional view, God is free to create because God is primordially and originally and necessarily Triune; on the revolutionary proposal, God is Triune because God decides to create. According to classical theology, God is necessarily Triune as Father, Son, and Holy Spirit but only contingently Creator and *incarnate* Son. But on the revisionist account, it looks as though the modal status of God-as-Triune and God-as-incarnate go together (as either contingent or necessary).

McCormack's response to van Driel is helpful in some ways, and we can follow his own summary by emphasizing the following points.

(BLM-1) There is no mode of being or existence in the triune life of God above and prior to the eternal act of self-determination in which God "constitutes" himself as "God for us" and, therefore, there is no such thing as an "eternal Logos" in the abstract. The Logos appears already in the immanent Trinity as the Logos *incarnandus* ... (thus) the Father never had regard for the Son apart from the humanity "to be assumed."[32]

(BLM-2) The eternal act in which God gives to himself his own being as Father, Son, and Holy Spirit and the eternal act in which God chooses to be God in the covenant of grace with human beings is *one and the same act*.[33]

---

[32] Bruce L. McCormack, "Seek God Where He May Be Found: A Response to Edwin Chr. van Driel," *Scottish Journal of Theology* 60:1 (2007), p. 66.
[33] McCormack, "Seek God Where He May Be Found," p. 66.

(BLM-3) The triunity of God is a function of divine election. To be sure, neither precedes the other chronologically. But it is God's act of determining himself to be God for us in Jesus Christ which constitutes God as triune.[34]

(BLM-4) While it is true that there is no act (or decision) without a subject, the identity of that subject may not be distinguished from the identity of God as constituted in the event in which God chooses to be God "for us" – because the being of the subject may not be distinguished finally from the act in which its being is given.[35]

And (BLM-5) There is no difference in content between the immanent Trinity and the economic Trinity ... The identity of both the *Logos incarnandus* and the *Logos incarnatus* is the same. The second person of the Trinity has a name and his name is "Jesus Christ" (the God-human in his divine-human unity).[36]

McCormack makes these points explicit. It is also important to note that what lies "behind" (or "beneath") these core affirmations is this fundamental conviction:

(BLM-0) Genuine knowledge of God is possible and actual only on the basis of God's revelation, which is ultimately found in the person of the God-human, Jesus Christ. Natural theology leads only to misinformation and ultimately to idolatry. Genuinely theological activity will be not only post-metaphysical but also anti-metaphysical.[37] Thus authentic theology will eschew abstract speculation and any claims to knowledge of God that are not based on God's revelation in Christ.[38]

---

[34] McCormack, "Seek God Where He May Be Found," p. 67.

[35] McCormack, "Seek God Where He May Be Found," p. 67.

[36] McCormack, "Seek God Where He May Be Found," pp. 66–67.

[37] E.g., McCormack, "Theses in Response to George Hunsinger," p. 122.

[38] Kevin Diller summarizes the concern in this way: "First, there is no hidden truth about God or God's being which is not revealed in Christ which, if known, would provide a deeper or more substantively different view of who God is. God doesn't have an unknowable essence or back-side which, if known, would adjust in any important way our knowledge of God." Therefore, "abstract metaphysical speculation – working only from generalized principles of human reason and experience, methodologically bracketing the historical particularities of God's acts – is not only doomed to failure, it is idolatrous in orientation." "Is God *Necessarily* Who God Is? Alternatives for the Trinity and Election Debate," *Scottish Journal of Theology* 66:2 (2013), p. 211. Stephen H. Webb notes that McCormack "consistently (and annoyingly) uses metaphysics and its related synonyms as pejoratives," *Jesus Christ, Eternal God: Heavenly Flesh and the Metaphysics of Matter* (Oxford: Oxford University Press, 2012), p. 332 n40.

(BLM-0) is at the root of McCormack's relentless drive to combat metaphysics and his resolute insistence on a properly theological ontology that is not dependent on metaphysics but is instead responsive only to the revelation of God in the person of Jesus Christ. Given (BLM-0), the employment of "classical metaphysics"—no matter how critically appropriated—is simply not a legitimate option for the theologian who is wholly and authentically Christian.[39] Doctrines of "classical theism" such as impassibility and divine simplicity are not tenable. Formulations of Christian doctrine that rely upon classical metaphysics must be re-conceived.[40] And, of course, the theological interpretation of the Bible is vital in the work of theology.

3.2.4 McCormack's Theological Exegesis

Accordingly, McCormack engages in theological exegesis as he seeks to show that his proposal is grounded in revelation. He judges that "one of Karl Barth's most significant contributions to exegetical theology lay in his recognition that passages like Col. 1:15–20; John 1:1–18; Heb. 1:2–4 and 1 Pet. 1:18–20 do not set forth the concept of a *logos asarkos* – in the sense of a true and genuine mode of being in the Son above and prior to the divine election."[41] McCormack follows Barth in his theological exegesis; he recognizes that "we are operating in the realm of *implications* when we seek to tease out the ontology implicit in the narrative," and he insists that this not only can but should be done.[42] With Barth, he argues that the New Testament depictions of Christ are not concerned with some shadowy unhuman or pre-human "Son" or *logos asarkos* but instead are centered on the particular and embodied human *Jesus Christ*. Typical is his handling of the Christology of Hebrews. Drawing from the *exordium* of Hebrews, he says that "it is one and same subject who was appointed, who makes purification, and then sits down."[43] As he explains

---

[39] McCormack is even sharply critical of Barth where he judges Barth to have been inconsistent in the rejection of metaphysics, e.g., *Orthodox and Modern*, pp. 211–212.

[40] E.g., McCormack, *Orthodox and Modern*, pp. 201–233 (especially p. 208 n18).

[41] Bruce L. McCormack, "With Loud Cries and Tears: The Humanity of the Son in the Epistle to the Hebrews," in Richard Bauckham, Daniel R. Driver, Trevor A. Hart, and Nathan MacDonald, eds., *The Epistle to the Hebrews and Christian Theology* (Grand Rapids: William B. Eerdmans Publishing Co., 2009), p. 59 n44.

[42] McCormack, "With Loud Cries and Tears," p. 59.

[43] McCormack, "With Loud Cries and Tears," p. 59.

The "Son" is not another or different subject than the subject who makes purification; he is the same subject viewed from a different angle. Structurally speaking, this is the logic of two "natures" – but it will not do to express that logic in terms of substance metaphysics. The distinction of a being in and for himself and a being for us is the distinction created by substance metaphysics, but it is not a distinction our writer was working with. Instead, he says simply, "The Son was appointed, and then he did this, and finally he did that." But it is one and the same subject of whom he speaks at every point in this narrative. Following the logic of this narrative, what we have to say is that the One through whom the world was made, the One who is the "exact imprint of God's very being" is not the "eternal Son" (if by that is meant a Son whose identity is abstracted from the humanity he would assume in the incarnation) but the Son whose identity is already established in that he is appointed heir of all things.[44]

This means that the "being of the Son is given in election." The "'eternal Son' has a name and his name is Jesus Christ."[45]

McCormack notes that "virtually any NT scholar" would deny that the "substance metaphysics of the ancient world is to be found in any of the NT writers," and he argues that it is such metaphysics that gives rise to the very Christological and theological problems that he is seeking to overcome (with Barth's help).[46] McCormack marshals the following considerations in favor of his view. First, he notes that the traditional reading of Hebrews 1 assumes a Trinitarian account that is not explicit in the passage. He specifically criticizes the work of John Webster at this point. As he describes matters, Webster holds that the Son is a "*Logos asarkos* whose identity is complete in itself, without reference to the humanity that he would assume in time," for the identity of the Son "consists in a relation to the Father which has been abstracted from the relation of the God-human in time and made to be its eternal and unchanging ground."[47] "The problem" with such an approach, as McCormack sees it, is that "the epistle has nothing to say about inter-trinitarian distinctions and the personal perfections of the divine persons to

[44] McCormack, "With Loud Cries and Tears," p. 59.
[45] McCormack, "With Loud Cries and Tears," p. 59.
[46] McCormack, "With Loud Cries and Tears," p. 60.
[47] Bruce L. McCormack, "The Identity of the Son: Karl Barth's Exegesis of Hebrews 1:1–4 (and Similar Passages," in Jon C. Laansma and Daniel J. Treier, eds., *Christology, Hermeneutics, and Hebrews: Profiles from the History of Interpretation* (New York: Bloomsbury T&T Clark, 2012), p. 160.

which they are alleged to give rise." Instead, the text is "ruthlessly silent on these points," and instead "all we are given in the epistle is the economic panorama."[48] To be clear, McCormack is not at this point saying that the traditional position (as represented by Webster) is wrong simply because it is not explicit in the text. Instead, as I understand him, he is making the case that the traditional view does not deserve anything close to the presumption of truth that is has received in some circles. It is not well-supported in the passages to which the traditionalists often appeal, and it is not impregnable. We can call this the "Lack of Grounding Objection" to the traditional view.

We can refer to his second argument as "The Naming Argument." McCormack observes that John and the author of Hebrews consistently refer to the Son as *Jesus Christ*. At first glance it may not seem obvious how this observation can be made into an argument; after all, a pro-Nicene traditionalist such as Webster can readily point out that this is hardly surprising and not at all unsettling for his position, for the New Testament texts in question are generally referring to the *incarnate* Son. But perhaps there is more to the pro-revisionist argument than initially meets the eye. Or perhaps the argument can be bolstered in a way that McCormack may not have considered. McCormack, at least so far as I can tell, seems to think of the name "Jesus Christ" as something like a "rigid designator." According to Saul Kripke's influential formulation, a rigid designator is a term that designates the same entity in all possible worlds (in which that entity exists).[49] Or, to put it a bit more precisely, the point is that "a designator d of an object x is rigid, if it designates x with respect to all possible worlds where x exists, and never designates an object other than x with respect to any possible world."[50] So if some d is the rigid designator of a necessarily existing object x, then d designates x in every possible world. On the other hand, if d is the rigid designator for some contingent object, then d designates that object in all possible worlds in which that object puts in an appearance. Applied to the case at hand, the proper name *Jesus Christ* is the rigid designator for the Son; it picks him out or designates him in all possible worlds in which the Son exists. There are no possible worlds in which there is a Son that is not Jesus Christ. The New Testament clearly refers to the Son as Jesus Christ, so, if that

[48] McCormack, "The Identity of the Son," p. 161.

[49] Saul Kripke, *Naming and Necessity* (Cambridge, MA: Harvard University Press, 1972), p. 48.

[50] Taken from a letter from Saul Kripke to David Kaplan, cited by Jason Stanley, "Names and Rigid Designation," in *A Companion to the Philosophy of Language*, Bob Hale and Crispin Wright, eds. (Oxford: Blackwell Publishing, 1997), p. 556.

proper name is a rigid designator, then it designates the Son in all possible worlds in which the Son has existence. And, as McCormack notes, the Son "has a name and his name is Jesus Christ." If this is the divinely revealed name of the Son, and if this name is a rigid designator, then there are no possible worlds where the Son exists but does not exist as Jesus Christ.

Third, and perhaps most important, is what we can refer to as "The Unity Argument." McCormack makes much of the link between priesthood and sonship in Hebrews. Following the exegesis of Richard Bauckham (while seeking to move beyond it theologically by insisting that we draw out the ontological implications of what is in the text), he points out that Hebrews teaches not only the enthronement and sovereignty of Jesus but also his priesthood. Thus Heb. 5:5 cites Ps. 2:7, which refers to the filial relation, along with Heb. 5:6 which cites Ps. 110:4 directly in reference to Jesus: "you are a priest forever according to the order of Melchizedek." McCormack sees here a link of "the Davidic coronation formula with entry into the eternal priesthood of Christ."[51] The point is not simply that Jesus Christ is the king while also being the high priest. That much is true, of course, but to stop there is to miss what is important. The salient point seems to be something more like this: the sonship, the sovereignty, and the priesthood are very closely and even inextricably related. The exact nature of this relationship is less than pellucid in McCormack's work, but it must be something in the neighborhood of necessity. Perhaps the claim is that these elements are coextensive and mutually entailing. Maybe it is stronger; perhaps these elements are not only coextensive but actually constitutive of one another. Either way, the upshot is plain enough: the filial, royal, and priestly aspects of the person and work of Christ are inextricably linked, and it is not possible to have one without the others. If the Son's filial relation is eternal and necessary, then so is his work as priest. If his sovereignty is somehow essential to him, then so is his priestly vocation. As McCormack sees things, if Bauckham's exegesis is correct, then it "requires us to conclude" that "Jesus Christ simply *is* the second person of the Trinity."[52] For the priesthood of Christ is nothing less than "eternal – and if eternal, then it too is included in the divine identity"; here "priesthood is made intrinsic to the divine identity."[53]

[51] McCormack, "With Loud Cries and Tears," p. 64.
[52] McCormack, "The Identity of the Son," p. 163.
[53] McCormack, "The Identity of the Son," p. 163.

3.3 Theological Analysis

3.3.1 Is It "Biblical?" Exegesis and Theology

At least one of Barth's contemporaries understood Barth along lines similar to McCormack. But Emil Brunner's reaction was negative: "No special proof is required to show that the Bible contains no such doctrine, nor that no theory of this kind has ever been formulated by any theologian."[54] Is Brunner right that the Bible contains no such doctrine? Or is McCormack right? Does a proper interpretation of the relevant biblical witness demand it? Is biblical teaching so much as suggestive of it, or at least consistent with it? Let us consider McCormack's arguments in order.

Turning to the "Lack of Grounding Objection," recall McCormack's insistence that the traditional view is read *into* rather than *out of* the text. As he says, the text (here, Hebrews, but also in John and Paul) is "ruthlessly silent" with respect to "inter-trinitarian distinctions."[55] He insists that the text deals only with the economy of salvation, and, while he is exercised to explore the implications of the biblical description of that economy, he is also adamant that the traditional view is not to be found in the text. By my lights, McCormack makes some important points here—but they are not decisive in favor of the revisionist account. At least three considerations are noteworthy. The first is that even if the defender of the sort of traditional view that is articulated by Webster readily (and, for that matter, perhaps even heartily) agrees with McCormack when he says that the full-blown pro-Nicene account is not spelled out in the text of Hebrews (or elsewhere), she need not think that this matters all that much. Since the case for the traditional view does not depend upon an explicit basis, and since the revisionist and the traditionalist alike can affirm this while also insisting that the implications of what is in the text are important, so far there is nothing to separate the revisionist from the traditionalist. Thus far, there is (methodological) concord. The second consideration is closely related. It is simply the observation that *neither* the traditionalist account nor the revisionist account can claim an easy victory from explicit biblical statements.

---

[54] Emil Brunner, *The Christian Doctrine of God, Dogmatics: Vol. 1*, translated Olive Wyon (Philadelphia: Westminster Press, 1949), p. 347, cited in Webb, *Jesus Christ, Eternal God*, pp. 235–236.
[55] McCormack, "The Identity of the Son," p. 161.

Neither depends on such an argument, and neither is fatally weakened by the lack of it. But, to be clear, McCormack's revisionist Christology and accompanying Trinitarian theology are nowhere spelled out in Scripture either. Again, to this point there is (or at least can be) methodological agreement. To the extent that McCormack's argument here is intended to serve as a "defensive" dialectical strategy (in "playing defense" against pro-Nicene arguments drawn from Scripture), to this point it might be judged successful. But if the revisionists were to wield it as an offensive weapon against the traditional account, then they would have more work to do. And here is where the third observation comes in to play: it may yet be the case that a pro-Nicene and even pro-Chalcedonian interpretation of key Christological passages in Hebrews (and other relevant texts) is the *best* overall interpretation. If we assume that the best overall interpretation is the most charitable one, and if we assume further that the most charitable interpretation is the one that offers hope of coherence, and then if we have good arguments that the pro-Nicene and pro-Chalcedonian readings offer a coherent account of the Christology and theology of Hebrews (and, *mutatis mutandis*, similar texts), then we may have good reason to conclude that the traditional interpretations are the best interpretations overall.[56] Indeed, some recent scholarship on Hebrews mounts such a case; Madison Pierce, for instance, argues that Hebrews gives us a window into intra-Trinitarian relations and communication.[57] But such considerations aside, my point here is simply that McCormack has not ruled out either the plausibility of such a conclusion or the possibility of good arguments for it. For present purposes, we can simply note that even if we judge McCormack's argument to this point to be successful as a defensive strategy (and thus admit there are no explicit "proof texts" for the traditional account of the identity of the Son as *logos asarkos*), it does not amount to a positive argument for his proposal.

Turning now to the "Naming Argument," several considerations seem relevant and important. I begin by simply noting that there are further complexities involved in the notion of "rigid designators." Beyond the

---

[56] Daniel Keating is convinced that Thomas Aquinas's overtly creedal interpretation of Hebrews "casts light on the text and helps to resolve genuine tensions within the letter itself," "Thomas Aquinas the Epistle to the Hebrews: 'The Excellence of Christ,'" in Jon C. Laansma and Daniel J. Treier, eds., *Christology, Hermeneutics, and Hebrews: Profiles from the History of Interpretation* (New York: Bloomsbury T&T Clark, 2012), p. 99. This is also the conviction of Thomas Joseph White, O. P., *The Incarnate Lord: A Thomistic Study in Christology* (Washington: Catholic University of America Press, 2015).

[57] Madison Pierce, *Divine Discourse in the Epistle to the Hebrews: The Recontextualization of Spoken Quotations of Scripture* (Cambridge: Cambridge University Press, 2020).

influential and basic account offered by Kripke, there are multiple theories.[58] If the revisionist were to take my suggestion and develop an argument along these lines, she would need to do so in a well-informed and careful way. The relevant point is simple: while this might be a promising way forward for the revisionist, there is work yet to be done. This brings us to the second consideration: however the development of the argument were to go (with respect to the philosophy of language and which precise account of rigid designators is adopted), it would need to proceed in a way that is not question-begging. It would need to address this question: Why not simply think of "Son" as the rigid designator? In other words, to function success-fully as a pro-revisionist argument, it would need to rule out the traditional view that the identity of the Son *as Son* (in relation to the Father) is necessary but that the incarnation is contingent. And it would need to do so while paying careful attention to the important metaphysical issues, complications, and entailments that are involved. Finally, even if it can show that "Jesus Christ" should be understood as the "rigid designator" (rather "the Son"), it would need to go further and demonstrate that this name is the rigid designator for *all the possible worlds in which the Son exists* rather than merely *all the possible worlds in which the Son is incarnate as human.* For the traditionalist could accept the latter—and without being moved from her traditionalism. I do not mean to suggest that the revisionist could not make such an argument. I only point out that it would need to happen—and has not yet been done. Unless and until it is, there is little here to persuade the traditionalist that her view is mistaken or problematic.

This is the case even if we accept McCormack's account of what "the name" is (and then try to bolster the case by appeal to the notion of a "rigid designator"). But perhaps to grant this much is to grant too much. For some important recent exegetical scholarship makes the case that "Jesus Christ" is *not* "the name" that is the appellation for the Son. These scholars argue that the name is the divine name. This is not, of course, to deny that the name of the incarnate Son is Jesus Christ. But it is to make the point that the author to Hebrews is concerned to show that the Son is above the angels—and indeed to be worshiped by them—precisely because the Son shares God's name. Peeler argues that the "only two vocatives" in the first chapter are addressed to the Son; the author cites Psalm 44 to "boldly" position God as addressing the Son as θεός, and the author cites Psalm 101 to have God

---

[58] For an introduction to the issues and an overview of the major options, see Stanley, "Names and Rigid Designation," pp. 555–585.

address the Son as κύριος.[59] This is, as Peeler points out, "not God and Lord, but Lord God, κύριος θεός, a designation for God in Israel's scriptures (Gen 2–4; Exod 34.14; Lev. 8.35; Josh. 7.19; Judg. 4.23)."[60] Richard Bauckham concurs: "the name that is so much more excellent than those of the angels must be the Hebrew divine name, the Tetragrammaton."[61]

McCormack's third argument is the most impressive and most important. The "Unity Argument" makes a case from the integrated nature of Christ's person and work as it is presented in Hebrews. So far as I can tell, McCormack actually has several considerations supporting his argument here. At one level, he is making the case from the eternality or everlasting-ness of Christ's priesthood. Heb. 5:6 tells us that Christ is a "priest forever, in the order of Mechizedek." McCormack concludes that if Christ's priesthood is "eternal, then it too is included in the divine identity"; here "priesthood is made intrinsic to the divine identity."[62] It is well known, of course, that αἰῶνα does not bring us anywhere close to a decisive case for timeless eternity. To conclude this would be to commit exegetical malpractice; the term simply means something like "age" more broadly and can readily be used to refer to everlastingness. Surely McCormack knows this, so this cannot be his argument. Instead of a lexical argument, the case seems to be a more broadly exegetical one. But here is where we must ask how it goes. Both the term itself and the immediate context are open to the suggestion that this refers to something that is forwardly everlasting but not backwardly everlasting, as something that simply has everlasting significance or that will not come to an end. McCormack could at this point admit this (of Heb. 5) but then direct us to Heb. 7:3 where the comparison of Jesus Christ to Melchizedek is strong and direct—and where Melchizedek is said to be "*without beginning* of days or end of life." To build too much on the linkage to Melchizedek would seem rather risky, for the identity of Melchizedek himself remains very shadowy and is much debated.[63] But even if the identity of Melchizedek is shadowy, the statement in Hebrews is significant,

[59] Amy Beverage Peeler, *You Are My Son: The Family of God in the Epistle to the Hebrews* (New York: Bloomsbury T&T Clark, 2014), p. 59.

[60] Peeler, *You Are My Son*, p. 59.

[61] Richard Bauckham, *Jesus and the God of Israel: God Crucified and Other Studies on the New Testament's Christology of Divine Identity* (Grand Rapids: William B. Eerdmans Publishing Co., 2009), p. 239.

[62] McCormack, "The Identity of the Son," p. 163.

[63] For a helpful discussion of Melchizedek in relation to Jesus, see Madison Pierce, *Divine Discourse*, pp. 104–114.

and it may be important for McCormack's argument. Gareth Cockerill maintains that the statement that "he remains a priest forever" is the "climax" of the first three verses of Heb. 7 (as μένει is the "main verb in the long Greek sentence that makes up vv. 1–3").[64] I take it that the salient point here is that Melchizedek, who is a priest forever, is "without beginning." So, by parity, Christ, who is also without beginning, is likewise a "priest forever." In response, however, the traditionalist can point out that Melchizedek's *priesthood* is not explicitly said to be "without beginning." Moreover, it is not even said to be αἰῶνα but instead is described as εἰς τὸν διανεκές.[65] So the linkage between Melchizedek and Jesus is not tight or relevant in every way, and, even if it were, this would not show that Christ's priesthood was eternal. It may indeed be forwardly everlasting—indeed this seems plain from the text. But such an affirmation neither equals nor entails the further claims that it is timelessly eternal or backwardly everlasting.

Even if we grant McCormack's account of an eternal priesthood, however, the heart of the issue is not temporality so much as it is modality. The most important question (for an analysis of McCormack's argument) is not "how long is Christ serving as priest?" Instead, it is "is the priesthood of Christ somehow 'intrinsic' to the Son's identity in the sense of being necessary or essential to him?" Here it is important to realize that statements such as "Christ's priesthood is eternal" or "Christ's priesthood is everlasting" are not equivalent to "Christ's priesthood is necessary to his identity" or "Christ is a priest in all possible worlds." Nor do the former statements entail the latter statements. For matters of modality are distinct from those of temporality. The modal status of a proposition is independent of temporal considerations, and it does not change with time.[66] Consider a proposition such as

(P) The Son serves as high priest from t1 to tn.

If (P) is true, then (P) is always true—whether or not it is necessarily true, and regardless of what the time stamp on t1 is. Note that (P) itself does not

---

[64] Gareth Lee Cockerell, *The Epistle to the Hebrews*, New International Commentary on the New Testament (Grand Rapids: William B. Eerdmans Publishing Co., 2012), p. 302.

[65] Albert Vanhoye argues that the difference here signals something about Melchizedek's priesthood that is less than the eternity or everlastingness that is used with reference to Christ, *Old Testament Priests and the New Priest According to the New Testament* (Petersham, MA: St. Bede's Publications, 1986), p. 153.

[66] See the discussion in Keith E. Yandell, *The Epistemology of Religious Experience* (Cambridge: Cambridge University Press, 1993), p. 360.

tell us anything about its modal status. So consider further the difference between

(P*) The Son serves as high priest from t1 to tn in all possible worlds

and

(P**) The Son serves as high priest from t1 to tn in some possible world(s) but not in all possible worlds.

For McCormack's exegetical argument to be wielded successfully in support of his revisionist proposal, it would have to make the additional step of arguing that (P*) (rather than (P**)) is the correct disambiguation of (P). Such an additional argument might come from metaphysical considerations (which would add a philosophical supplement to an exegetical argument and thus make connection to (BLM-0) rather more tenuous). Or perhaps it might be supplied by further exegesis. But until we have good reason to think that (P*) is right, McCormack's argument gives no support to his proposal.

In addition to the argument from eternity, however, McCormack seems to be arguing from the relation of Christ's person to his work. He sees the link between Christ's filial relation and priestly vocation as a kind of "package deal." As it is not possible for Christ to serve as priest (in the functions and to the ends described in Hebrews) without being the Son, so also it is not possible for him to be the Son without also serving as priest. McCormack is not alone in seeing such strong links and tight connections. Cockerill says that "high priesthood is intrinsic to the Son's identity as both all-sufficient Savior and Revealer."[67] Similarly, Amy Beverage Peeler concludes "Jesus is Son and therefore he is Priest."[68] As she puts it pithily: "If Son, then Priest." So what are we to make of this argument?

---

[67] Gareth Lee Cockerill, *The Epistle to the Hebrews*, New International Commentary on the New Testament (Grand Rapids: William B. Eerdmans Publishing Co., 2012), p. 77. Compare F. F. Bruce, *The Epistle to the Hebrews*, revised edition, New International Commentary on the New Testament (Grand Rapids: William B. Eerdmans Publishing Co., 1990), p. 29; Harold Attridge, *The Epistle to the Hebrews: A Commentary on the Epistle to the Hebrews* Hermeneia (Philadelphia: Fortress Press, 1989), p. 25; Peter O'Brien, *The Letter to the Hebrews* Pillar New Testament Commentary (Grand Rapids: William B. Eerdmans Publishing Co., 2010), p. 35.

[68] Amy Beverage Peeler, "If Son, Then Priest," in Caleb T. Friedeman, ed., *Listen, Understand, Obey: Essays on Hebrews in Honor of Gareth Lee Cockerill* (Eugene: Pickwick Publications, 2017), p. 96.

What has been shown; what has been demonstrated exegetically? And what is implied by what has been shown? Note that when Cockerill says that "high priesthood is intrinsic to the Son's identity," he adds that it is the Son's "identity *as both Savior and Revealer.*" To take this as supporting evidence for McCormack's proposal would be to over-read the statement. Cockerill does not say that priesthood is intrinsic to the Son's identity *simpliciter*; instead he refers to the Son *qua* the Son's vocation and mission. It is to the Son as Savior and Revealer that he refers. Thus what he says is consistent with both the traditionalist account and the revisionist proposal. Consider Peeler's statement: "If Son, then Priest." This could be taken as support for the revisionist view, but, again, that would be to read too much into it. The statement "If Son, then Priest" surely represents the teaching of Hebrews well, but it does not resolve the issue before us. Here is why: the statement does not claim that the Son's priesthood is somehow *necessary*. In fact, it makes no claim about the modal status of Christ's vocation. Of course we know that the Son's filial relation is compossible with his priestly vocation. This much is plain from the teaching of Hebrews. And of course we are in a position to know that this is *possible*—if something is actual, then it is possible, so if Christ's priesthood is actual, then we can be certain that it was possible. But nothing about the actuality of the Son's priesthood implies the necessity of it. Again, Peeler's statement neither claims nor entails the conclusion "If Son, then necessarily Priest"—and if it did, it would not represent the teaching of Hebrews. For as Peeler concludes, although "the author of Hebrews views Jesus's filial identity as integral to his priesthood, he does not present his priesthood as a vocation automatically entailed by his identity as Son."[69] "If Son, then Priest" yields "If Son, then *possibly* Priest" (perhaps as a rather trivial entailment), but it does not give us "If Son, then *necessarily* Priest."

In our evaluation of the "Unity Argument" to this point, we have been proceeding by granting much that McCormack assumes about the proper exegesis of Hebrews. But these assumptions themselves are less than secure. Many contemporary Hebrews scholars do not share McCormack's assumption that the Son's priesthood is eternal.[70] Nor do they think that it is intrinsic to his divine filial relation. David M. Moffitt observes that Hebrews 7 portrays Jesus as priest *although* he is Son (rather than *because*

---

[69] Peeler, *You Are My Son*, p. 124.
[70] See the helpful survey of views by R. B. Jamieson, *Jesus's Death and Heavenly Offering in Hebrews* (Cambridge: Cambridge University Press, 2019), pp. 4–25.

he is Son) and that in Heb 5:8–10 he *became* the source of salvation.[71] He notes that 2:17 says that Jesus became a high priest (ἵνα...γένηται... ἀρχιερεύς).[72] Moffitt argues extensively that the role of high priest is not given by birth (as Jesus is not a Levite), that such a role comes only as Jesus is "perfected" through his suffering death, and that he performs the functions of high priest precisely as the *resurrected and ascended* Son who continues to make atonement for his people. For while he is "on earth, Jesus's tribal lineage prevents him from serving as a priest," and this is obtained by "being transformed such that he has an enduring life."[73] He makes the case that "the royal son became high priest," and "careful attention to the writer's use of Ps 110:4 and the argumentation of Heb 7 supports the hypothesis that Jesus's resurrection is foundational for Jesus's high priestly status."[74] Moffitt concludes that there is a definite temporal moment when the high priestly duties of the Son began: "It was *after* Jesus was perfected that he became the source of everlasting salvation for all those who obey him, *being at that time* appointed by God high priest according to the order of Melchizedek."[75] Pierce agrees: "Christ is 'made perfect' when he returns to life," and "through his indestructible death, he is qualified for priestly ministry (7:16, 24)."[76] Jamieson also concurs; he argues that "Jesus was appointed high priest at his entrance to heaven, on the basis of his being made perfect by resurrection."[77]

Putting this together, we can conclude that McCormack's exegetically based case for his proposal is less than successful. Although it goes against the grain of much contemporary Hebrews scholarship, perhaps it can be bolstered (I have indicated one such way that this might be done with respect to the "Naming Argument"). But unless and until further work is done to bolster it, sound exegesis of Hebrews (and, I would argue, similar texts) does not demand the revisionist account. At the very least, we must consider the case unproven. On the other hand, there are exegetical

[71] David Moffitt, "It Is Not Finished: Jesus' Perpetual Atoning Work as the Heavenly High Priest in Hebrews," in Jon C. Laansma, George H. Guthrie, and Cynthia Long Westfall eds., *So Great A Salvation: A Dialogue on the Atonement in Hebrew* (New York: Bloomsbury T & T Clark, 2019), p. 160.

[72] Moffitt, "It Is Not Finished," p. 162 n14.

[73] David M. Moffitt, *Atonement and the Logic of Resurrection in the Epistle to the Hebrews* (Leiden: Brill, 2013), p. 213.

[74] Moffitt, *Atonement and the Logic of Resurrection*, p. 200.

[75] Moffitt, *Atonement and the Logic of Resurrection*, p. 197, emphasis original.

[76] Pierce, *Divine Discourse*, p. 197.

[77] Jamieson, *Jesus's Death and Heavenly Offering in Hebrews*, p. 25. Cf. R. B. Jamieson, "When and Where Did Jesus Offer Himself? A Taxonomy of Recent Scholarship on Hebrews," *Currents in Biblical Research* 15:3 (2017), pp. 338–368.

considerations that might count against McCormack's proposal. These should be taken seriously as well.

3.3.2 Does It Hold Together? Concerns about the Coherence of the Revisionist Proposal

Moving forward, we begin by picking up the aforementioned concerns about coherence and internal consistency. As we have seen, several prominent critics charge McCormack's view with incoherence. What are we to make of these criticisms? Before moving forward, it is important to note that all parties in these debates care about coherence. The "traditionalist" interpreters of Barth charge the "revisionists" with incoherence, and McCormack is quick to return the compliment. For instance, he says that Hunsinger's "reading of Barth's doctrine of God is fundamentally incoherent," that Hunsinger "finds himself on the horns of a dilemma that he fails to resolve," and that the "resultant incoherence is only deepened by his attempt to use Jüngel's interpretation of Barth to invest his own reading with authority."[78] Neither side wants to admit incoherence, and both sides will weaponize charges of incoherence and wield them against the other. So no one is in a position simply to wave off such concerns or to dismiss them as only the "use of classical philosophy and metaphysics." But what are we to make of the worries about internal consistency and coherence with respect to McCormack's revisionist proposal? As it turns out, there are several areas of concern.

One such area has to do with McCormack's statements about divine freedom. Put together, these statements are rather puzzling. Consider the following claims:

(Thesis 9) As a description of the being of God in the act of election, the freedom of God is a freedom for self-determination and, indeed, self-*limitation* and suffering for the sake of human beings. It is God's lordship over all things, including his own being. In that God chooses to be God for us in Christ, he is giving himself the being he will have for all eternity.[79]

---

[78] McCormack, "Theses in Response to George Hunsinger," pp. 116–118.
[79] McCormack, "Theses in Response to George Hunsinger," p. 135.

Taken in the context of his overall account of Trinity and election, this is not surprising. But now compare these statements offered in explanation of the thesis:

> (Thesis 9B) "God's freedom does not consist in a choice between alternatives," for "such a conception, however venerable it may be, is far too anthropomorphic" and at any rate "requires 'time' for deliberation in order to be meaningful";[80] and

> (Thesis 9C) "God's freedom is finally the freedom to exist – or not to exist. The opposite of the determination to be God in the covenant of grace is not a determination to be God in some other way; rather, it is the absence of such a determination, which would mean choosing not to exist."[81]

As it stands, (9B) is a bit ambiguous. Interpreted in a broader sense, (9B) denies that alternative possibilities are relevant for divine freedom (whether or not they exist). Read more narrowly, (9B) denies that there *are* alternative possibilities. Which way should we take it? The context makes it fairly clear that the narrower reading of (9B) is the proper interpretation, for McCormack also says that the "idea of counterfactual possibilities is rendered *unreal* (i.e., lacking in reality)."[82] But the only plausible way to read (9C) is as an affirmation of alternative possibilities. "To exist" and "not to exist" are contraries. Thus they are alternatives. Whatever exactly it means to say that God might choose not to exist is a matter that we will revisit in due course, but at this point I note that it appears—at least initially—that McCormack's account of divine freedom is of dubious coherence.

Another area of interest, one that is related, concerns the revisionist account of the humanity of Christ. As we have seen, McCormack places significant weight on the distinction between the Logos *incarnandus* and the Logos *incarnatus*. He employs this distinction in order to insist that the Logos was always to-be-incarnate but not eternally or everlastingly incarnate. However, Stephen Webb wants to know why McCormack does not go further and maintain that the humanity of Jesus Christ is eternal. Webb's own view is similar to that of McCormack—but it is even more thoroughgoing. Like McCormack, Webb is convinced that the Logos just *is* the man Jesus Christ; the second person of the Trinity is identical to the incarnate

[80] McCormack, "Theses in Response to George Hunsinger," p. 135.
[81] McCormack, "Theses in Response to George Hunsinger," p. 136.
[82] McCormack, "Theses in Response to George Hunsinger," p. 135.

God-human that is named Jesus Christ. But unlike McCormack, Webb is prepared to take the full implications of this view with complete and thorough seriousness. As he sees things, this means that we should affirm that the humanity of Jesus is eternal. He recognizes that McCormack refuses to take this step, for McCormack says that "the human nature (body and soul) of Jesus came into existence at a particular point in time, in history."[83] It is here that Webb pushes McCormack. Jesus Christ simply is the incarnate Son, the God-human. The humanity is part of his identity as such; it constitutes the person of the Son. Webb asks: "How could that name be eternal if the person to whom it refers is not?"[84] Webb sees McCormack's assertion that "as we look at Jesus Christ we cannot avoid the astounding conclusion of divine obedience," and he presses the issue: "When we look at Jesus Christ, we see more than just obedience. We also see his body. Indeed, it is that body that makes his act of obedience possible, so why doesn't McCormack attribute it to the Trinity as well?"[85] Webb thinks that there is an inconsistency here that hobbles McCormack's attempt at theological revolution, and he concludes that McCormack is left with "a very weak version of full, personal pre-existence of Jesus Christ."[86]

3.3.3 The Issue of Divine Freedom

McCormack's statements raise some fascinating and important issues with respect to divine freedom. As we have seen, van Driel worries that McCormack's proposal comes to the same end as Hegelianism; even if they come via different routes, the two theories entail the same conclusion. The issues are complicated, and some careful analysis may be helpful here.

If I understand it correctly, McCormack's proposal seems to be positing that the modal status of *God is Triune* and *God is incarnate* is the same. And since *God is incarnate* entails *God creates (a world with humankind)*, then creation shares modal status with *God is Triune* and *God is incarnate as the man Jesus Christ*. The upshot of this is that if God's existence as Trinity is necessary, then so is God's existence as incarnate and thus as Creator, but if God's existence as Trinity is contingent, then so is God's existence as incarnate and thus as Creator. If God's electing choice-to-be-incarnate-and-Triune

---

[83] McCormack, "Grace and Being," p. 96.   [84] Webb, *Jesus Christ, Eternal God*, p. 238.
[85] Webb, *Jesus Christ, Eternal God*, p. 332 n40.
[86] Webb, *Jesus Christ, Eternal God*, p. 239.

is logically prior to God's Triunity, then God's Triunity is necessary if and only if God's electing choice is necessary. And, of course, if election is contingent, then God's Triunity would be contingent as well. A contingent choice cannot produce a necessary being. A contingent choice would produce a contingent being. On the other hand, a necessary action would produce a necessary result. So it seems that the modal status of God-electing and God-Triune would be the same.

McCormack's proposal, as it stands, is rather ambiguous. It could be interpreted as maintaining that God's Triunity and creation-incarnation are necessary, or it could be taken to claim that God's Triunity and creation-incarnation are not necessary but instead are contingent. Interpreters both sympathetic and critical take McCormack's proposal in various ways. Kevin Hector says that according to revisionism God's "self-determination is necessary while triunity is contingent."[87] But van Driel disagrees; "on this proposal," he avers, "triunity is a necessary implication of the choice made in election; election being essential to God (and therefore necessary, if God is necessary), so is triunity."[88] Given the ambiguity of McCormack's statements and the fact that his theology is still developing, neither interpretation is implausible. But both open into yet more options. If we take the revisionist proposal as a necessity-positive claim, then we are left with two major interpretive options. It may be that *some* possible world with creation of humanity is necessary, or it may be that *this* possible world is necessary. On the other hand, if we take it as a contingency-positive claim, then we have the following options: either "God" could decide to be non-creative and non-incarnate and thus non-Triune, or God could decide against election and thus cease to exist. It is not clear just how to take McCormack's position. Some of his interpreters and defenders have pressed some distance into these alternatives, but a closer look is warranted.

3.3.3.1 Necessitarian Versions

Let us begin with the necessitarian readings.[89] If this is correct, then God is necessarily Triune. God is also necessarily the one who is creative and

---

[87] Kevin Hector, "God's Trinity and Self-Determination: A Conversation with Karl Barth, Bruce McCormack and Paul Molnar," *International Journal of Systematic Theology* 7:3 (2005), p. 251.

[88] van Driel, "Karl Barth on the Eternal Existence of Jesus Christ," p. 54 n39.

[89] A critic who interprets McCormack along these lines is Paul D. Molnar, *Divine Freedom and the Immanent Trinity: In Dialogue with Karl Barth and Contemporary Theology* (Edinburgh: T&T Clark, 2002), p. 63: "the order between election and triunity cannot be logically reversed without in fact making creation, reconciliation and redemption necessary to God."

incarnate; indeed, it is the decision to be God-with-us in creation and incarnation that establishes or "constitutes" God as the Triune Father, Son, and Holy Spirit. This much is held in common by necessitarian readings, but from here things diverge. Consider the version that says that *this* possible world is necessary. We can refer to this version as

($\Box$1) It is necessary that God be creative, incarnate, and Triune, and it is further necessary that God so constitutes his Triune-and-incarnate identity by creating (or, more precisely, "actualizing") this possible world.

McCormack is emphatic that it is *this* electing Act that constitutes God's being. Further, he insists that "it is in his history that [the Son] is constituted the 'person' he is."[90] Accordingly, some commentators interpret the revisionist proposal as an affirmation of ($\Box$1). Scott R. Swain concludes that this is McCormack's most mature account of divine freedom: "if we have correctly understood McCormack's view of God's freedom…then it appears that God's freedom *ad extra* consists in his ability to enact his will to create *this world and this world alone*."[91]

The revisionist need not hold that the world is made necessary for God by any external constraint or coercion. She need not admit that God is unfree in this sense. The revisionist can deny that there are any forces, either personal agents or impersonal forces that are independent of God that cause or compel God to act in this way. She can insist that God has "freedom of volition" (Hector/Diller), but this is compatible with God's decision being determined by factors that are internal to God. In other words, this is basically a compatibilist notion of divine freedom. Some of what McCormack says coheres nicely with this view. He judges Barth to have "come to the very edge of the Hegelian identification of the Son of God with a human being," and he applauds this move by Barth.[92] He holds that God is indeed free from any "external constraint or conditioning."[93] And, as we have seen, he denies that God's freedom should be thought of as "choice between alternatives."[94] So this surely seems like a possible and plausible rendering of McCormack's revisionism.

---

[90] McCormack, *Orthodox and Modern*, p. 224.
[91] Scott R. Swain, *The God of the Gospel: Robert Jenson's Trinitarian Theology* (Downers Grove: InterVarsity Academic, 2013), p. 222.
[92] McCormack, *Orthodox and Modern*, p. 242.
[93] McCormack, "Theses in Response to George Hunsinger," p. 135.
[94] McCormack, "Theses in Response to George Hunsinger," p. 135.

But is such an account of freedom enough? Sure, God does what God wants to do, and God does so in the absence of any external constraint or compulsion. Nonetheless, in point of fact it is not possible for God to do anything other than what God in fact does. This has some weighty consequences. At one level, it entails a version of panentheism. Definitions of panentheism are varied, and surely there are different kinds of panentheism. But one common thread running through many accounts of panentheism is the commitment to the notion that creation is necessary to God. We might call this *modal* panentheism. Clearly, this interpretation of McCormack's view is panentheistic in this sense.

But however one judges panentheism, there is a far more serious worry. It is this: the threat of modal collapse. Since on this view we are affirming necessity, let us assume that God's existence is necessary; God exists, that is, in all possible worlds. Let w^* stand for this world, the actual world. Let A stand for God's act of actualizing w^*. Now consider this argument:

(1) If there is no liberty of alternatives for God, then God is not free to refrain from A;

(2) God's freedom does not consist as "choice between alternatives"; there is no liberty of alternatives for God;

(3) Therefore, God is not free to refrain from A (from 1 and 2);

(4) If God is not able to refrain from A, then it is not possible that w^* not be actualized;

(5) Therefore, it is not possible that w^* not be actualized (from 3 and 4);

(6) If it is not possible that w^* not be actualized, then the actualization of w^* is necessary;

(7) Therefore, w^* is both possible and necessary.

A possible world is a maximally consistent state of affairs. If some *maximally consistent* state of affairs is necessary, then it seems that is the only one that is possible. But then we have collapsed possibility into necessity. And if possibility collapses into necessity, then we have modal collapse. Another word for modal collapse is better known among theologians: fatalism. God may not be constrained to create by any combination of external factors, but it is nonetheless true that God's existence entails our own existence. If God exists, then you and I exist. This world—in all its detailed minutiae and with its full measure of sin and suffering—exists necessarily. It could not be otherwise, even for God. Since God exists, then it is not possible that I not wear a blue shirt on the fourth Monday of the fourth month of my fortieth year, and it is not possible that Hitler and his minions torture and kill even one less innocent victim. Nothing could be different than it is—even for God.

Alternatively, suppose that we take the other necessitarian view. We can summarize this as:

(□2) It is necessary that God be creative, incarnate, and Triune, but the divine decision to be so is free in the sense that this is possible and feasible in more than one world.

On this account, the creation of *some possible world with human creatures* is necessary for God—but the options for God are not constrained to *this* world. God could not be God without *some* creation, and this creation would have to include humans (for the possibility of incarnation as human). But God could have made a world without Genghis Khan (and, of course, without his sixteen million or so male descendants); God could have made a world without elephant seals or armadillos but with unicorns and orcs instead. In other words, given the reality of his own nature, the creation of some world that includes humans (for the sake of incarnation) is inevitable for God, but God could have actualized a human-containing world other than w^*. So God's essence or nature makes creation necessary, but God has some alternatives with respect to what God creates. Diller offers something like this as a possible way forward for McCormack. In a lucid and analytically precise discussion of these issues, he registers an important concern: "If creation is a necessary consequence of God's essence... then doesn't that make the divine being dependent on human beings? Does not this introduce an extraordinarily unseemly ontological dependence of the Creator on the creation? And what has become of preserving the graciousness of God's action with the affirmation that 'God would be God without us?'"[95] Diller argues that nothing about this view would violate the Creator-creature distinction. Nor does it make God causally dependent on the creation. He also distinguishes between libertarian divine freedom and divine freedom from external constraint, and he claims that God's having freedom from external constraint "with respect to God's decision to create is sufficient to preserve God's liberty of volition."[96]

---

[95] Diller, "Is God *Necessarily* Who God Is," pp. 216–217.
[96] Diller, "Is God *Necessarily* Who God Is," p. 217.

It is not clear, however, that the revisionists will want to endorse this alternative. For it is not yet obvious that it does not violate (BLM-0). If God could have done differently than God in fact did, then is there not some conceptual space where God might have done something different? And if God's being is constituted by what God *does* with respect to creation, then would not a world even somewhat different raise the worry that God would have been—and thus could have been—somewhat different? Even some of McCormack's sympathizers and defenders are concerned that he has left open the possibility of a hidden deity. As Diller says, granting logical priority to election over the Trinity "appears to create space for a hidden God or naked will behind the revealed God."[97] Hector expresses a worry similar to that of Diller when he says that the problem "is that McCormack's move appears to make God's self-determination into an abstraction: whereas Barth identifies God's self-determination in the concrete interaction between Father, Son, and Spirit, McCormack abstracts this self-determination from this relationship and makes it into a 'thing-in-itself...God's decision to be God-with-us becomes an 'absolute will' rather than God's eternal, triune act."[98] Moreover, it is not apparent that the revisionists *should* want to endorse it. For even if this route avoids the fatal trap of modal collapse, it is still left with the commitment to panentheism. Here the distance from Barth grows farther.

3.3.3.2 Non-Necessitarian Versions

Some of McCormack's statements lend themselves to a non-necessitarian view. For instance, he insists that divine freedom is "finally the freedom to exist – or not to exist."[99] This suggests a rejection of necessitarianism that is quite emphatic. McCormack endorses Barth's rejection of the notion that "It is an intrinsic impossibility that He should not be or should be other than He is."[100] At least two non-necessitarian versions are possible for the revisionist who holds that God's self-constituting decision of election and God's Triunity share modal status. One is rather more radical than the other.

---

[97] Diller, "Is God *Necessarily* Who God Is," p. 218.
[98] Kevin Hector, "God's Triunity and Self-Determination," p. 258.
[99] McCormack, "Theses in Response to George Hunsinger," p. 136.
[100] McCormack, "Theses in Response to George Hunsinger," p. 133. Here he references Karl Barth's *Church Dogmatics*, translator G. W. Bromiley, eds., G. W. Bromiley and T. F. Torrance (Edinburgh: T & T Clark, 1956), II/1, p. 307.

The less radical version is this: there is an ontologically primordial divine being who exists necessarily but who contingently decides to be the incarnate-and-Triune-God-for-and-with-us. We can refer to this as

(~□1) God's existence is necessary, but God's decision to be creative, incarnate, and Triune is contingent rather than necessary, thus it is possible that God exists without being Triune-and-incarnate-and-creative.

Some of what McCormack says would seem to cohere with this position. Responding to Molnar, McCormack insists that "God need not have created this world; God might have chosen to create a different world or to have created no world at all."[101] He says that the statement "*God* would be God without us" is a "true statement and one that must be upheld at all costs if God's grace is to be truly gracious."[102] In his response to van Driel, McCormack says that "the only thing that is absolutely necessary for God is existence itself."[103] He warns us against considering this in abstraction "from the decision in which God gives to himself his own being," and while we are well-advised to heed his warning and take his advice (on his view, it really *is* the case that God *did* give himself this being), this does not change the substantive claim made: the only thing that is absolutely necessary for God is existence itself. If this is true, and if it is also true that election is logically more basic than Triunity, then we might well come to the position: This deity exists necessarily but contingently decides to be the God known in and through Jesus Christ as the Triune God.

Several steep challenges face this proposal. First, we wonder why we might think that it is true. The words of Brunner again come to mind: "No special proof is required to show that the Bible contains no such doctrine, nor that no theory of this kind has ever been formulated by any theologian."[104] If any theological proposal seems speculative, surely it is this one. So if McCormack is right that theological speculation is bad, then this proposal is awful.

Moreover, not only is it untethered from Scripture (and tradition), it is unhinged in a way that provokes the very worries that seem to motivate McCormack to take his revisionist position. If any theology posits a "hidden

---

[101] McCormack, *Orthodox and Modern*, p. 297.
[102] McCormack, *Orthodox and Modern*, p. 274.
[103] McCormack, "Seek God Where He May Be Found," p. 67.
[104] Emil Brunner, *The Christian Doctrine of God*, p. 347, cited in Webb, *Jesus Christ, Eternal God*, pp. 235–236.

deity" lurking "somewhere behind the back of Jesus," then surely this is it. This deity is almost entirely unknown and even unknowable.

This may be slightly too quick. Perhaps there are *some* things that we can deduce about such a being—but if this is so, then matters get worse. This deity has some attributes or properties, and logically must if these are to (logically) precede the divine decision to be Triune-incarnate-creative. As van Driel notes, "One would think that at least there has to be divine willing, and also divine power."[105] But at some (logical) point, this deity would be not-incarnate and thus not-Triune. And if this is right, then this deity is not *homoousios* with the Triune God. This deity has the property of necessary existence, and, according to modal logic, has this property necessarily.[106] And since this deity has the property of necessary existence with *de re* necessity, then it has the property essentially. But the incarnate-and-Triune-God-for-and-with-us has the properties *being Triune* and *being incarnate* only contingently. If it has these properties contingently, then it has them non-essentially. And a God who is not essentially Triune is not the God of historic creedal orthodoxy. Defenders of the revisionist proposal will be quick to remind us that we are talking only about *logical* priority and that all notions or presumptions of temporality must be banned altogether at this point. Fair enough, but the central modal and metaphysical—and thus *theological*—issues are nonetheless at stake.

The more radical version is suggested by McCormack's statement that real freedom for God is the freedom whether or not to exist at all. Where the other non-necessitarian version holds that the deity who makes the electing decision to be incarnate and Triune only has to exist but could exist in some other way and could have been "constituted" differently, another non-necessitarian version could maintain that this deity has two basic options: exist as God-Triune-and-incarnate or cease to exist. We can refer to this version as

(~□2) It is neither necessary that God exists or that God is creative, incarnate, and Triune, but if God exists then God is creative, incarnate, and Triune. God has real options and alternative possibilities, but they boil down to this: Trinity or nothing.

---

[105] van Driel, "Karl Barth on the Eternal Existence of Jesus Christ," p. 54.
[106] At least on S4 ($\Box p \Rightarrow \Box\Box p$) and S5 ($\Diamond p \Rightarrow \Box\Diamond p$).

In other words, there are possible worlds in which God fails to exist. But all possible worlds in which God exists are worlds in which God elects to be, and thus is, creative, incarnate, and Triune.

This version sits uncomfortably with some of McCormack's statements, but it coheres well with his assertion that divine freedom is "the freedom to exist – or not to exist."[107] Taken along the lines of the current version of non-necessitarianism, we would take this to mean "the freedom to exist-with-and-for-humankind-as-incarnate-and-Triune – or not to exist at all." In other words, it is either the Triune God of the Christian faith as revealed in Christ or deicide. This is (or perhaps *was*) a real option, but it is the only one.[108] The ultimate and sober truth is this: Trinity or nothing.

An interesting parallel to this can be found in recent work in analytic philosophy of religion. Keith E. Yandell stands as a clear and shining example of an analytic theologian who rejects perfect being theology (at least of the common, Anselmian type). Yandell contrasts what he labels "plain theism" with "Anselmian theism." For the Anselmian theologian, God exists necessarily; God exists in all possible worlds, and God exists as necessarily maximally excellent and good in all possible worlds. God is the greatest conceivable being, the one who is maximally excellent as well as necessarily existent. There are no possible worlds in which God commits sin, for God is, strictly speaking, both necessarily existent and necessarily *good*. So on *Trinitarian* Anselmian theism, all divine persons are necessarily good. And on *incarnational* Trinitarian Anselmian theism, the divine person who is now incarnate for us is necessarily good as human and divine. Yandell recognizes that a broadly Anselmian view is dominant historically; he knows that this is the default position in the Christian tradition. Nonetheless, he diverges from this tradition, and in place of Anselmianism he offers "plain theism." According to plain theism, "*being divine*, Judeo-Christianly con-strued, includes being omnipotent and omniscient and morally perfect."[109]

---

[107]   See also his sympathetic discussion of John Zizioulas's claims that "the being of God is not an 'ontological necessity,'" McCormack, "Theses in Response to George Hunsinger," p. 133 n22. See further John D. Zizioulas, *Being As Communion: Studies in Personhood and the Church* (Crestwood, NY: St. Vladimir's Seminary Press, 1993), p. 41.

[108]   Scott R. Swain says that "I do not take divine nonexistence as a real possibility in McCormack's metaphysical scheme," *The God of the Gospel*, pp. 221–222. Instead, he takes it as a *per impossible* statement (p. 222). I do not know if this does full justice to McCormack's intentions. But if it does, then it is a vacuous claim. As the system of modal logic known as S5 makes plain, if something is possible, then it is really possible and even necessarily possible.

[109]   Keith Yandell, "Divine Necessity and Divine Goodness," in Thomas V. Morris, ed., *Divine and Human Action: Essays in the Metaphysics of Theism* (Ithaca: Cornell University Press, 1988), p. 315.

Of course perfect being theology agrees with this. The divergence between plain theism and perfect being theology can be seen, however, in what it means to be "morally perfect." For the perfect being theologian, moral perfection equals or at least entails necessary moral goodness. For the plain theism theorist, however, this isn't at all obvious—perhaps *moral* perfection isn't even consistent with necessity. After all, the defender of plain theism argues, there are good reasons to think that moral responsibility demands robust freedom. We shouldn't misunderstand the claim of plain theism here: it surely *isn't* the claim that God *is* less than morally perfect, it *is* the claim that God's moral perfection is logically contingent rather than necessary. Nor should we draw the wrong conclusions about plain theism. As Yandell explains, plain theism does not entail that divine goodness isn't completely *stable*:

> For all that, if [plain theism] is true, deicide is not something to worry about. For if God can know the future – in particular, can know His own future choices – He can know whether He will ever choose to sin or not. Suppose He knows He will not. So deicide will not occur. Suppose He knows he will. Then He now knows that He will sin in the future, and does nothing now to prevent that inelegance, and so is not morally perfect even now, and so has committed deicide already. So if God exists at all, and deicide is a sin, then deicide will never occur. Whatever reason we have to think that God does exist, we have the same reason to think that He will not self-destruct, whether or not [Anselmian theism] is true.[110]

Perhaps there is a similar case to be made for this version of the revisionist proposal; maybe there is something analogous here. If one adds omniscience and then can find a way to make moral goodness coextensive with being Triune-and-incarnate (along the lines of McCormack's revisionism), then perhaps one could mount an argument that we can deduce, from the fact that God *is* incarnate-with-and-for-us-and-Triune, that God will always be this way. For if God knows the future (at least his future) exhaustively, then God knows if he will in any way fail to be morally good by being God-with-and-for-us-as-incarnate-and-Triune. And if God were to know that he would fail in this way, then God would already be complicit and thus already

---

[110] Yandell, "Divine Necessity and Divine Goodness," pp. 315–316. This summary of Yandell's proposal is taken from my, *An Invitation to Analytic Christian Theology* (Downers Grove: InterVarsity Academic, 2015).

in a state of such failure. Accordingly, if we can now know that God is not failing morally, then we could know that God will never fail morally.

At any rate, again we might be troubled by the questions that haunt the other version of non-necessitarianism: why believe that this is true? Is this not speculative, and perhaps even wildly so? If theological speculation really is a form of idolatry, then is this not ideological Baal-worship? And we are left with the specter of a deity behind the back of the Triune God revealed in and through Jesus Christ. If that is an unwelcome implication, then the lesson to be learned is that this is not a good theological option for the revisionist.

3.3.4 The Identity of The Decider

These considerations raise a question of particular interest and real importance. Just who or what is this deity that makes the decision? What is its identity? Again, the revisionist proposal is underdeveloped, but several options emerge.

Before moving forward, however, it may help to get clear on the meaning of identity. I take it that what the revisionists are after here is nothing short of numerical identity, for merely qualitative "identity" surely won't do, and at any rate settling for merely qualitative identity would certainly violate (BLM-0). Thus understood, identity is *reflexive, transitive,* and *symmetric.* Because any object x is identical to x, identity is reflexive. If x is identical to y and y is identical to z, then, because identity is transitive, x is identical to z. And, as symmetric, if x is related to y, then of course y is related to x. Identity is an equivalence relation that satisfies the law of the Indiscernibility of Identicals:

(InId) For any objects x and y, if x and y are identical, then for any property P, x has P if and only if y has P.[111]

Of course, (InId) requires the appropriate world (and time) quantifiers to account for transworld identity (and temporal change), but the basic point should be clear.[112] With this clarification about identity in mind, let us

---

[111] $(\forall x)\ (\forall y)\ [x = y \Rightarrow (\forall F)\ (F(x) \Leftrightarrow F(y))].$

[112] Anything having to do with temporality is bracketed in light of McCormack's repeated insistence that the Trinity-constituting act of election is not temporal. For an overview of

return to the question of the identity of the electing deity. Just who is this deity?

3.3.4.1 The Father

One such option is that this is the Father or proto-Father. On this reading, the subject who elects is the one who "becomes" (though, once again, logically but non-temporally on McCormack's view) the Father. This subject can hardly be said to be the Father already, because the Father is Father only in relation to the Son (just as the Son is Son only in relation to the Father). So until there is a Son, there is, strictly speaking, no Father. So this would be a proto-Father. McCormack notes that "one prominent strand of ancient reflection on the Holy Trinity" holds that "the 'Father' alone is *autotheos* and because that is so, he is the *fons deitatis* and the *fons et erigo* where the being of the other two 'persons' of the Trinity is concerned."[113] McCormack says that he can "walk hand in hand with this line of reflection for a considerable stretch" (departing from this by insisting that there is only one eternal event rather than two).[114] Further, he says that while we can speak of "*God's* act of self-determination to be God 'for us,'" nonetheless it is more accurate and therefore better to "speak of the 'Father' as the subject who gives himself his own being in the act of election."[115] So this is not implausible as an interpretation of the revisionist proposal.

But what are we to make of it? A couple of issues deserve a closer look. First, note that McCormack says that the "'Father' gives himself his own being." But at most this could only be *partly* true, for the proto-Father must already be in the possession of some attributes and abilities in order for this to be the case. Minimally, the proto-Father must have a set of decision-making abilities and their concomitant properties. After all, *he* is the one who makes the call. Moreover, the proto-Father has abilities to make the decision mean something; he has the power not only to want something to be the case but also to make it the case. Presumably, then, the proto-Father has significant power and knowledge attributes—if not omniscience and omnipotence then something very close. Answers to other questions are less

---

relevant issues of modal quantification, see Michael J. Loux, "Introduction," in Michael J. Loux, ed., *The Possible and the Actual: Readings in the Metaphysics of Modality* (Ithaca: Cornell University Press, 1979), p. 42.

[113] McCormack, "Seek God Where He May Be Found," p. 67 n17.
[114] McCormack, "Seek God Where He May Be Found," p. 67 n17.
[115] McCormack, "Seek God Where He May Be Found," p. 67.

clear. For instance, does the proto-Father have the attribute of love prior to the decision that constitutes Trinity, incarnation, and creation? Of course the defender of revisionism will be quick to remind us that we are not talking about temporally located or sequenced events. Fair enough, but the questions of (modal) logic still loom large. So, again, does the proto-Father have the attribute of love (logically) prior to the Trinity-constituting decision? Is divine love contingent? Is it (*de re*) necessary and thus essential? Is it essential to the constituted Trinity (as one would assume) but not essential to the proto-Father? Such questions remain open, but they are important enough to deserve further consideration by the proponents of the revisionist account. The upshot is this: it isn't exactly right to say that *the Father* gives himself his own being; instead we should conclude that the proto-Father uses certain attributes that are already in his possession to configure or constitute deity in one particular way.

Moreover, the identity of the proto-Father in relation to the Father is unclear, and there is some cause for concern. For if the identity of the Father is constituted by his relation to the Son (as is central to the creedally orthodox tradition and as I assume McCormack maintains), then the proto-Father is without a Son prior to election. But then the Father and the proto-Father cannot be identical (given InId), for the Father has a necessary property—his relation to the Son—that the proto-Father does not have. And, of course, the proto-Father has a property not had by the Father, for the proto-Father is the one who elects Triunity while the Father (simply by virtue of being the *Father of the Son*) finds himself so constituted within the Trinity. The troubles deepen if we go with either of the non-necessitarian readings. Consider:

(8) If the proto-Father has different identity conditions than the identity conditions of the Father, then the proto-Father is not the same entity or person as the Father;

(9) The proto-Father has different identity conditions from those of the Father;

(10) Therefore the proto-Father is not the Father.

On the non-necessitarian readings, the proto-Father could exist without being the Father. Even on the more radical version, the proto-Father exists "long" enough to will himself out of existence, and thus would exist apart from the Son. But the Father is Father only in relation to the Son. Shorn of the appearances of temporality, it is possible that the proto-Father be Father and possible that the proto-Father not be Father. But since the identity of the Father is constituted only in relation to the Son, it is not possible for the Father to be Father without the Son.

On McCormack's view, it may indeed be the case that "there is no difference in content between the immanent Trinity and the economic Trinity," but there indeed is a difference between the Father and the proto-Father. This is a conclusion that would seem problematic not only for the tradition but also for McCormack, for he wants to agree with Barth that "God's being is *absolutely* his willed decision; not additionally, not subsequent to a being above and prior to that decision, but *absolutely* his willed decision."[116]

Another area of concern is perhaps more serious. Recall McCormack's observation that there is a strand of older theology that holds that only the Father is, strictly speaking, *autotheos*. Only the Father exists *a se*, and the Son and the Holy Spirit have their divinity derivatively. McCormack concurs.[117] He is certainly correct that there is this strain within the tradition. In the tradition of Reformed theology, this teaching has been the occasion for some controversy. Some theologians in the broadly Reformed tradition held that only the Father is *autotheos*; their view is that the Son receives his very divinity from the Father. Jacob Arminius, for example, will allow that the Son is *autotheos* as an affirmation that the Son is truly and wholly God, but he also rejects any view according to which the Son has an essence held in common with the Father but not coming from the Father.[118] Arminius holds this view rather than the more common Latin or Western position. As Richard A. Muller summarizes it,

> In the traditional Western model, as argued by Peter Lombard and ratified in the Fourth Lateran Council, the divine essence neither generates nor is generated; rather the person of the Father generates the person of the Son – with the result that the Son, considered as to his sonship, is generated, but considered as to his essence is not. Or, to put the point another way, there is no essential difference between the Father and the Son, the only difference being the relation of opposition, namely, the begottenness of the Son.

---

[116] McCormack, "Seek God Where He May Be Found," p. 74.

[117] McCormack, "Seek God Where He May Be Found," p. 67 n17. He demurs, of course, with the traditional account of the Trinity and the God-world relation found in this older theology.

[118] See further Keith D. Stanglin and Thomas H. McCall, *Jacob Arminius: Theologian of Grace* (New York: Oxford University Press, 2012), pp. 86–90.

The Son, therefore, has all of the attributes of the divine essence, including aseity.[119]

So in what appears to have been the majority or received view, other theologians held that the Son is also *autotheos* with respect to his divinity but only receives his personhood-constituting relationship from the Father. In other words, for the majority position (within the Reformed tradition), aseity is rightly attributed not only to the Father but also to the Son (and Spirit). Their distinct personhood is constituted by their relationships to one another; after all, the Father is only the Father in relation to the Son, and the Son is Son only in relation to the Father. But the divinity of the Father is not a different divinity than the divinity of the Son—as it would be if the Father alone had the attribute of aseity while the Son and Spirit did not have it.[120]

McCormack pretty clearly seems to land on the side of Arminius in this debate. But doing so raises the familiar worries. If aseity is rightly to be understood as essential to God, then we are faced with the following argument:

(11) If the Father has the attribute of aseity and the Son does not, then the Father and Son are not *homoousios*;

(12) The Father has the attribute of aseity, but the Son does not;

(13) Therefore, the Father and the Son are not *homoousios*.

This has long been the subject of debate, and it is no stretch to think that both the revisionists and the more traditionally minded defenders of the position held by Arminius will have more to say. But the challenge should be obvious: if the Father has essential properties or attributes of divinity that the Son and Holy Spirit do not have, then the Father is not of the same essence as the Son and Holy Spirit and thus not *homoousios*.

3.3.4.2 The Son

Interestingly, Webb reads the revisionist proposal as positing the Son as the one who elects. He says that McCormack "attributes the decision to be an electing God to the second member of the Trinity, in accordance with

---

[119] Richard A. Muller, *Post-Reformation Reformed Dogmatics, Volume 4: The Tri-unity of God* (Grand Rapids: Baker Academic Press, 2003), p. 88.

[120] Brannon Ellis, *Calvin, Classical Trinitarianism, and the Aseity of the Son* (Oxford: Oxford University Press, 2012).

Barth's argument that Jesus Christ is both the elector and the elected."[121] Webb is both puzzled and frustrated by this proposal:

> But if election determines God's triune identity, then the Son can be said to beget himself. That is, by deciding to be the electing God, the Son determines himself to be begotten of the Father. This follows if one assumes that the Trinity is the product of election and election is determined by the Son. The resulting definition of God is too circular to try to sort out.[122]

He observes that McCormack at least recognizes the appearance of a problem, and he also notes that rather than address the problem head-on, McCormack falls back on a claim about "our inability as humans to comprehend the meaning of an eternal decision."[123] Our real problem is our tendency "to think all too anthropomorphically."[124] Webb pushes back: if we follow Barth's lead and begin "by identifying God with the electing and the elected Jesus Christ, [we] cannot think otherwise than anthropomorphically."[125] If we really receive God's revelation as found in and as the man Jesus Christ, then we not only can but indeed *should* embrace anthropomorphism. If God is self-revelatory by taking the very form of humanity, then the proper response is to think of God in this way.

Consider McCormack's statement that humans are unable to "comprehend the meaning of an eternal decision." This may be true (I don't have arguments against it), but it is not exactly relevant to the point. For one thing, one need not *comprehend* something (in the sense of full and complete understanding) to truly be able to *apprehend* it (in the sense of having an incomplete but nonetheless meaningful and secure grasp of it). If comprehension of things divine were required for genuine knowledge of divinity, then no one other than God would have any knowledge of God. Thus the only appropriate type of theology would be ectypal theology, and no creature is up to that standard. For only an omniscient being can fully comprehend God. But there is no good reason to think that ectypal theology is the only theology that is possible. More importantly, the notion of the time—or lack thereof—of a decision is not the main issue. Of course it is the case that discussions of time and eternity are both important and very difficult, and of

[121] Webb, *Jesus Christ, Eternal God*, p. 239.
[122] Webb, *Jesus Christ, Eternal God*, p. 239.
[123] Webb, *Jesus Christ, Eternal God*, p. 239, quoting McCormack, "Grace and Being," p. 104.
[124] McCormack, "Grace and Being," p. 104.
[125] Webb, *Jesus Christ, Eternal God*, p. 239.

course it is the case that things get more complicated and troublesome for the revisionist account if we adopt a view of divine temporal everlastingness over timeless eternity, but that is not the most central issue here. What we are interested in here—again explicitly following McCormack's lead and trying to do justice to his proposal as it stands—are concerns about the (modal) *logic* (concerns that are independent of issues of time and eternity).

Webb despairs that the view is simply "too circular to try to sort out." But let us linger long enough to see some challenges that face it. Two of these are now familiar. Consider:

(14) If the Son has the property of being constituted as Son by a relationship to the Father but the proto-Son does not, then the Son has identity conditions which are different from those of the proto-Son;

(15) If the Son has identity conditions which are different from those of the proto-Son, then the Son is not the same entity (or "person") as the proto-Son;

(16) Therefore, if the Son has the property of being constituted by a relation to the Father but the proto-Son does not, then the Son is not the same entity (or "person") as the proto-Son;

(17) On this interpretation of the revisionist proposal, the Son has the property of being constituted as Son by a relationship to the Father, but the proto-Son does not (as it is logically prior to the Father-Son relationship);

(18) Therefore, on this interpretation of the revisionist proposal, the Son is not the same entity (or "person") as the proto-Son.

Suppose that the foregoing problem can be resolved. Another problem arises. Consider further what happens if we maintain that aseity is an essential divine attribute and then adopt a non-necessitarian version of the revisionist account:

(19) if the proto-Son/Son has the property of aseity and the Father does not, then the Father and Son are not *homoousios*;

(20) the proto-Son/Son has the property of aseity, but the Father does not;

(21) Therefore, the proto-Son/Son and the Father are not *homoousios*.

In sum, this approach faces challenges as steep and difficult as the view that the one who elects is the Father.

3.3.4.3 The Decider

As we have seen, not only is there ambiguity with respect to this key claim of McCormack, there is also support for understanding this to be a claim about the Father *and* there is reason to think that this is a claim about the Son. Well, maybe there is a sense in which it is both—although not either exactly. Maybe the electing entity is neither the Father nor the Son per se, but is instead something that somehow becomes both Father and Son (and, of course, Holy Spirit). This electing entity can simply be called *The Decider*. Perhaps it is "first" (again, in McCormack's logic-only sense of "first") either impersonal or unipersonal, but in the electing act it becomes a Trinity of persons. Maybe it does so through a process of fission, or perhaps it does so in some other way.[126]

It seems starkly obvious that if any version of the revisionist proposal runs afoul of (BLM-0), then surely this is it. If any theology has a deity that exists (logically) "behind" Jesus, then this is it. If theological speculation is conceptual idolatry, then we are in even deeper trouble, for with this proposal we are moving beyond intellectual Baal-worship to ideological Molech-worship. Accordingly, we will not linger long here, but it is also important to recognize that the now-familiar objections will also land with force here. On the non-necessitarian versions, The Decider clearly has different persistence and identity conditions than does the Trinity. For according to (~□1) and (~□2), The Decider exists necessarily (at least long enough to be able to will itself out of existence), while the Trinity only exists contingently. It is obvious that the Trinity and The Decider are not *homoousios*, and thus we have at least two gods.

3.3.5 Some Final Observations

Responding to van Driel, McCormack admits that "it is true that there is no act (or decision) without a subject"—and then attempts to ward off potential objections and concerns by asserting that "the identity of that subject may not be distinguished from the identity of God as constituted in the event in which God chooses to be God 'for us' – because the being of the subject may not be distinguished finally from the act in which its being is given."[127] What

---

[126] See the proposal of Peter Forrest, "Divine Fission: A New Way of Moderating Social Trinitarianism," *Religious Studies* (1998), pp. 281–297.

[127] McCormack, "Seek God Where He May Be Found," p. 67.

are we to make of this claim? Is it successful as a rejoinder? We might first simply ask what it means. When McCormack says that "we may not distinguish," is he making an epistemological claim or is he making an ontological claim? Are we unable to distinguish simply because of our limitations and inabilities, or are we unable to distinguish because there is nothing distinguishable? In other words, are matters simply too cloudy from our side? Or is the "being" that is "given" and the "act" that gives identical? Is the act indistinguishable from the being *because* they are identical? If McCormack's claim is only that it is an epistemological barrier, then it is not easy to see how it can serve as a statement of theological ontology. Since theological ontology is what McCormack is after, it seems that it is not merely an observation about the limits of our knowledge but instead is a claim about the sober truth of the matter (truth that we can and should know).

The interpretive options surveyed all face challenges, but some of these challenges are much more daunting than others. Unfortunately, however, what seems to be the most plausible interpretation is also one of the most problematic. The most plausible rendering seems to be ($\Box$1) (with ($\sim\Box$2) as less likely but not implausible).[128] And McCormack's rejoinder (to van Driel)—which asserts that the Act of electing *this* world is identical to the (Triune) Being that is given to God in that Act—makes matters worse rather than better. If the Act of electing or choosing *this* world is identical to the Being of God, then, given (InId), all properties possessed by the Act must also be possessed by the Being. And all properties possessed by the Being must also be possessed by the Act. So not only are we left with the conundrum of how it might be that the Act is Triune *before* the Being is constituted as Triune, we are also faced with the conclusion that *this* world is entailed by God's Triune existence. So *this world* is essential to God. And this amounts to nothing short of modal collapse.

Perhaps the revisionist will simply shrug and dismiss all this as "metaphysical speculation." Maybe she will hand-wave these concerns away while rejecting them as wrong-headed and even as idolatrous. But this would be unfortunate, for the analysis offered here tries to gain clarity about the options and the prices involved with each. I do not intend this analysis as any kind of a

---

[128] McCormack's commitment to ($\Box$1) seems especially clear in his statements in "The Being of God as Gift and Grace: On Freedom and Necessity, Aseity and the Divine 'Attributes,'" Kantzer Lectures in Revealed Theology (2011), available at henrycenter.tiu.edu/resource/the-being-of-god-as-gift-and-grace-on-freedom-and-necessity-aseity-and-the-divine-attributes.

knock-down argument; where I have made criticisms it is to warn the revisionists from taking these routes or at least to alert them to the weaknesses that attend both the general proposal and the various disambiguations of it. Although I am not sanguine about the fortunes of the revisionist proposal and, candidly, think that it is both unmotivated and deeply mistaken in some ways, I neither say nor imply that the difficulties cannot be addressed, the concerns ameliorated, or the problems resolved. While I think that this kind of revisionist proposal needs careful theological analysis, I offer this exercise in hopes that it will be helpful for defenders and detractors alike.

Moreover, it would be especially unfortunate for the revisionist to dismiss this analysis as wrong-headed or idolatrous for at least two reasons. First, McCormack himself constantly talks of "logic" and "logical priority" (which he contrasts with temporal priority) as well as "being" and "identity" along with "essence" and "act." To make any sense at all of his arguments and claims, we simply must think with the tools that we have. If he has better (i.e., distinctly *theological*) accounts of logic and identity that are directly taught by Jesus Christ (or that actually and obviously are implied by the revelation of God in Christ), then let him share these with us. Until then, surely it is not wrong to use our best tools to think with him. Thus when he talks about logic and necessity, it is hardly unreasonable to use modal logic in an effort to understand (and thus either clarify, defend, or criticize the claim under consideration). Second, McCormack has already engaged in some analytic arguments of his own. Recall his rather scathing criticisms of Hunsinger; note especially how he charges Hunsinger with "incoherence." Charges of incoherence do not arise or find force in an intellectual vacuum. Instead, they presuppose, rely upon, and employ several fundamental notions in logic and metaphysics. If a view is incoherent (at least in the context in which McCormack makes the charges), then it is contradictory. More completely, it is false *because* it is contradictory. Apparently, something that is contradictory (and thus incoherent) is necessarily false for McCormack, for he labels positions and supporting arguments as "incoherent" without going on to show how or why that makes them problematic. But this only works if we rely on logical principles such as the "law of non-contradiction" and metaphysical notions such as identity. In other words, the revisionist who rejects out of hand the kind of analysis offered here would be making a case that is self-referentially incoherent. She would be criticizing her critics for using a set of conceptual tools that are said to be unacceptable for theology—but then using the very tools she rejects to criticize her own critics. She would be hoist on her own petard.

So where does this leave us? Well, as we have seen, the various interpretive options are fraught with difficulties and will no doubt continue to face challenges, and the version that seems to be the most plausible interpretation is also the among the most problematic.

3.4 Conclusion

McCormack's revisionist proposal is both intriguing and bold. I take it to be a developing proposal, one that is being adjusted and refined as arguments and counter-arguments move forward. I offer these reflections and arguments with the hope that they stimulate and enable further change, correction, and development. Aware that McCormack wants nothing to do with "classical" substance metaphysics, I have tried—much like Diller and Hector—to bring some contemporary analytic resources to the project.[129]

Accordingly, in this chapter I first surveyed the revisionist proposal and the contemporary debate that it has ignited. I then probed the exegetical foundations of McCormack's proposal; here I noted several shortcomings and pointed to areas of remaining work for the revisionists. I then explored issues relevant to the overall (internal) coherence of the proposal, and I raised some theological concerns about the proposal. It should be obvious that I think that these theological concerns are serious, and they deserve equally serious consideration. At this point I find the positive case for the revisionist account to be underwhelming, and I find the worries and objections to it to be powerful. But I do not mean to suggest that these objections cannot be met, but they stand in the way of broad acceptance of McCormack's fascinating proposal.

---

[129] For contemporary introductions to the "classical" or "scholastic" tradition, see Edward Feser, *Scholastic Metaphysics: A Contemporary Introduction* (Heusentamm: Editiones Scholasticae, 2014), and David S. Oderberg, *Real Essentialism* (New York: Routledge, 2007).

4

The Submission of Christ

4.1 Introduction

The author of Hebrews tells us that Jesus Christ did not exalt himself (5:5).
Instead, we are told that

> In the days of his flesh, Jesus offered up prayers and supplications, with
> loud cries and tears, to him who was able to save him from death, and he
> was heard because of his reverence. Although he was a son, he learned
> obedience through what he suffered. And being made perfect, he became
> the source of eternal salvation to all who obey him, being designated by
> God a high priest after the order of Melchizedek   (5:7–10).

This fascinating passage is both rich in insight and intriguing. It raises many
interesting interpretive and theological questions. Central to this passage is
the statement that Jesus Christ was obedient. The obedient subordination of
the Son is an issue that is the subject of intense debate in contemporary
Trinitarian theology and Christology; surprisingly, however, Hebrews 5 has
not figured significantly in those debates.

In what follows, I offer a brief exercise in the theological interpretation of
Scripture. This means different things in different contexts, so let me be clear
about what I mean: theological interpretation of Scripture seeks to interpret
the Bible theologically; it looks, that is, to see what the Bible teaches about
God (and all else as it is related to God). It does so in respectful dialogue with
the insights of modern and contemporary biblical studies, and it also seeks
to learn from the deep and broad Christian tradition of exegetes and
theologians. Accordingly, in this study we look closely for a proper understanding of the biblical witness to the submission and subordination of the
Son. We do so in close conversation with two important theologians:
Thomas Aquinas and Karl Barth. While both theologians seek to understand
the subordination of the Son in accordance with creedal orthodoxy, their
positions are importantly different. In what follows, I will offer a summary
of their views, outline some important criticisms, and then ask what

Analytic Christology and the Theological Interpretation of the New Testament. Thomas H. McCall,
Oxford University Press (2021). © Thomas H. McCall. DOI: 10.1093/oso/9780198857495.003.0005

Hebrews 5 contributes directly to these discussions. But first, however, it will be helpful to make a few preliminary observations about the text.

4.2 Hebrews 5:7-10: Some Initial Observations

This fascinating passage raises many interesting questions: what are we to make of the reference to the "days of his flesh,"[1] especially in light of the orthodox Christian commitment to the continuing incarnation (and thus humanity) of the Son?[2] To what do the "loud cries and tears" refer; is this a reference to the prayer in Gethsemane (Mark 14:32-42),[3] is it a reference to the cry of derelicition of the Son from the cross (Matt 27:43; Mark 15:34),[4] or

---

[1] Karl Barth holds that these "days" refer to his passion and especially to his death, *Church Dogmatics* III/2, trans. G. W. Bromiley, eds. G. W. Bromiley and T. F. Torrance (Edinburgh: T&T Clark, 1956), p. 562. He also thinks that these extend into the present, *Church Dogmatics* IV/3, p. 395. Thomas Aquinas puts the emphasis on the "flesh" here; he says that "flesh is taken for the entire human nature" (*tota natura humana*), *Super Epistolam B. Pauli ad Hebraeos Lectura*, translated as *Commentary on the Letter of Saint Paul to the Hebrews*, trans. F. R. Larcher, eds. J. Mortensen and E. Alarcon (Lander, WY: The Aquinas Institute for the Study of Sacred Doctrine, 2012), p. 113.

[2] I take these "days" to be a reference to his incarnate earthly career; his life on earth. See the discussion in Albert Vanhoye, *Structure and Message of the Epistle to the Hebrews* (Rome: Editrice Pontificio Instituto Biblico, 1989), p. 158. At any rate, the use of σαρξ in Hebrews does not carry the negative connotations that it sometimes does in Pauline theology.

[3] Karl Barth is convinced that this is a reference to Gethsemane. Indeed, he says that it is an "insufficiently noticed" commentary on Gethsamane, *Church Dogmatics* III/2, p. 337, cf. *Church Dogmatics* IV/2, pp. 95, 250. Aquinas is likewise certain that Gethsemane is in view here, e.g., *Hebrews*, p. 114. Commentators as diverse as F. F. Bruce, P. E. Hughes, and H. Orton Wiley are certain that Gethsemane is in view. See F. F. Bruce, *The Epistle to the Hebrews* (Grand Rapids: William B. Eerdmans Publishing Co., 1964), pp. 98–100; P. E. Hughes, *Commentary on the Epistle to the Hebrews* (Grand Rapids: William B. Eerdmans Publishing Co., 1977), p. 182; H. Orton Wiley, *The Epistle to the Hebrews* (Kansas City: Beacon Hill Press, 1959), pp. 181–183. On the other hand, scholars such as David deSilva (who thinks that passages from 2 and 3 Maccabees are more likely), Harold Attridge, and William Lane deny that this is so obvious. See David DeSilva, *Perseverance in Gratitude: A Socio-Rhetorical Commentary on the Epistle "to the Hebrews"* (Grand Rapids: William B. Eerdmans Publishing Co., 2000), pp. 190–191; Harold W. Attridge, *The Epistle to the Hebrews* (Minneapolis: Fortress, 1989), p. 148; William L. Lane, *Word Biblical Commentary, Hebrews 1–8* (Nashville: Thomas Nelson, 1991), p. 120. Gareth Lee Cockerill says that the "reference to Gethsemane is suggestive without being definitive," and while noting that "the pastor could have made such a reference unmistakable had he so desired," he concludes that "it is better to see this entire verse as a depiction of the utter dependence upon God that characterized the Son's earthly life and came to its climax in Gethsemane and on the cross," *The Epistle to the Hebrews*, NICNT (Grand Rapids: William B. Eerdmans Publishing Co., 2012), p. 244.

[4] Karl Barth connects this closely to the cry of derelicition, e.g., *Church Dogmatics* I/1, p. 386; *Church Dogmatics* I/2, p. 158. John Calvin and P. E. Hughes are among those who opt for both Gethsemane and the cry of derelicition. See John Calvin, *The Epistle of Paul the Apostle to the Hebrews and the First and Second Epistles of St. Peter*, trans. William B. Johnson, eds. David W. Torrance and Thomas F. Torrance, p. 64.

just what?[5] What are we to make of the statement that he was heard "because of his reverence" (5:7)? What is it to be a "high priest after the order of Melchizedek" (5:10)? And so on; there is no shortage of compelling questions here.

Along with such intriguing questions that arise in reading this text, however, we can also see that the passage makes some important affirmations. Indeed, the text does so with clarity and force. Several of these stand out as especially important for our discussion. First, we know that the Son was obedient. Jesus Christ "learned obedience through what he suffered" (v. 8). This theme is powerful in Hebrews (especially 10:7, 9). Of course, this teaching is by no means unique to Hebrews. Philippians 2:5-11 tells us that the Son was "in the form of God" but did not count equality with God as something to be grasped or held (v. 6). Instead, the Son became human and took upon himself "the form of a servant" (v. 7). He "emptied himself" and "humbled himself," and in so doing became obedient "to the point of death, even death on a cross" (v. 8). Moving beyond Paul, Jesus himself says that "I do not seek to please myself but him who sent me," (John 5:30); that "I do nothing on my own but speak just what the Father has taught me" (John 8:28), and that "the Father is greater than I" (John 14:28). So this is not a point that is unique to Hebrews, but it is important to see that it is very clear here. The Son really was obedient.

Second, the Son *learned* (ἔμαθεν) obedience (v. 8). This does not mean that he was ever *disobedient*. We should not assume that the options here are limited to merely *obedience* and *disobedience*, for someone could be *nonobedient* without being either obedient or disobedient. One person may stand in relation to another in which the options are either obedience or disobedience. So a soldier who enlists in the military and serves under a commanding officer must either be obedient or disobedient. But before he comes into this relationship—before, that is, he enlists—he is neither disobedient nor obedient. Before his enlistment he is merely nonobedient, and what makes the difference is the change that occurs. So we should not over-interpret this passage. The text does not tell us that the Son was ever disobedient, nor should we assume that he was. In fact, Hebrews tells us explicitly that the Son was "without sin"—even though he was truly tempted (4:15). But nor does it tell us that he was always obedient. It simply does not say that. So we should not over-interpret this passage or import assumptions

---

[5] Aquinas connects this to another of Christ's statements from the cross: "Father, into your hands I commit my spirit" (Luke 23:46), *Hebrews*, p. 114.

into it, but neither should we fail to see this salient point. What the text does say is clear enough, and it is important: the Son *learned* obedience.

Third, the Son learned obedience *through suffering* (v. 8). The learning (ἔμαθεν) comes via suffering (ἔπαθεν). The learning process is thus in the "days of his flesh" (ἐν ταῖς ἡμέραις τῆς σαρκός); it occurs during his earthly sojourn (v. 7). The obedience referred to in this passage is coupled with the incarnate Son's experience of suffering; it is not something that is said to be true of the Son eternally, nor is it said to be intrinsic to the identity of the Son or his relationship to his Father. Whatever we might learn about the obedience and subordination of the Son from other passages, and whatever we might conclude about it theologically, what is clear in this passage is that the Son learned obedience through suffering.

Fourth, this passage shows us that he learns obedience *as Son* (v. 8). He does not leave or abandon his filial relation to learn obedience—indeed, how could he do so? Instead, it is precisely *as Son* that he learns this obedience through suffering. As Cockerill points out, "Christ's sonship did not cease while he was learning 'obedience.' When the pastor speaks of the human Son he is always referring to the eternal Son who has assumed humanity."[6] The suffering does not establish the Sonship; the force of the "although" (καιπερ) is concessive here. Nor does it even serve to demonstrate it (cf. 12:3-11). But neither does it negate it. Accordingly, for Hebrews obedience is not inimical to the filial relation. Jesus Christ learns obedience through suffering, and he does so precisely *as Son*.

Fifth, the process of learning obedience through suffering is closely related to the high priestly work of the Son. Cockerill is right when he says that "the Son has been set apart for a fully effective priesthood through complete obedience," and "this offering of total submission to God unto death is his sacrifice of priestly consecration."[7] The "loud cries and tears" are the prayers of the Son who lived and died *for others*. Jesus Christ has been called or designated a high priest by God (v. 10), and it is in this capacity that he both learns obedience through suffering and becomes the cause or source (αἴτος) of eternal salvation for all who obey him (v. 9). As a high priest, he acts not on his own behalf but on behalf of others (5:1; cf. 2:17), thus it is for others that he prays and for others that he learns obedience through suffering. His work is not for himself, for he is holy and pure in his innocence (7:26). His work is not for himself, because he has no need of

---

[6] Cockerill, *Hebrews*, p. 247. [7] Cockerill, *Hebrews*, p. 240.

such work (7:27; 10:4, 10). What he does is on behalf of others. And what he does is enough; it is final. "This doing of God's will is the sacrifice that does away with all previous sacrifices."[8] The Son learns obedience while suffering to be the source of our eternal salvation; he learns obedience not in place of our obedience but so that we can be obedient too (v. 9). As Cockerill concludes, "By his obedience Christ makes their obedience possible."[9]

4.3 Karl Barth and Thomas Aquinas on the Obedience of the Son

4.3.1 Karl Barth on the Eternal Subordination of the Son

Karl Barth is, of course, well aware of the straightforward New Testament statements that speak to the subordination, submission, or obedience of Jesus. After all, Jesus himself says that "the Father is greater than I" (John 14:28). Barth is also surely well aware of the traditional distinction between what might be called *functional* or *economic* subordination, on one hand, and *ontological* subordination on the other hand. But while he clearly rejects Arian and Socinian views, he is reticent to avail himself of the traditional distinction. Instead, he thinks that submission or subordination belongs to the very nature of the Trinity. He sees the "dignity of Jesus, the Lordship of Jesus and the superiority of Jesus" as real but also as "basically different and subordinate compared to that of the Other who is properly called $\theta\epsilon$os."[10] He goes on to say that "what is beyond question is that the $\kappa\acute{\nu}\rho\iota$os Iσous $X\rho\iota\sigma\tau\acute{o}$s is separate from and subordinate to $\theta\epsilon$os $\pi\alpha\tau\grave{\eta}\rho$."[11] While these statements are somewhat short of finally decisive (Barth is here referring to the Son *as incarnate*), he further offers a ringing affirmation of the view that this subordination is more than merely functional within what is sometimes referred to as the "economic" Trinity. For Barth says that we must "affirm and understand as essential to the being of God the offensive fact that there is in God Himself an above and a below, a *prius* and a *posterius*, a superiority and a subordination."[12] To be clear, Barth speaks here of something that is "essential to the being of God," and it is obvious that he holds to a kind of hierarchy within the Trinity. The Son simply *is* the one who is obedient; the

---

[8] Cockerill, *Hebrews*, p. 242.   [9] Cockerill, *Hebrews*, p. 445.
[10] Barth, *Church Dogmatics* I/1, p. 385.   [11] Barth, *Church Dogmatics* I/1, p. 385.
[12] Barth, *Church Dogmatics* IV/1, pp. 200–201.

Son is the one "who is himself this act of obedience."[13] For "according to the New Testament, it is not the being of the man Jesus which has this character" of obedience.[14] No, "on the contrary," in the New Testament it is the Son of God who is described as the servant.[15] Thus the Son is obedient "not accidentally and incidentally... But necessarily and, as it were, essentially."[16] Indeed, Barth highlights the element that he labels "the most offensive fact of all"; this is the fact that there is "a below, a *posterius*, a subordination that... belongs to the inner life of God."[17] The Triune God is "both a First and a Second, One who rules and commands in majesty and One who obeys in humility. The one God is both the one and the other."[18]

It is worth noting that not all so-called "Barthians" agree with him on this point. Thomas F. Torrance, for instance, takes a very different approach both in affirming the full equality of the Son with the Father and in refusing to concede that the subordination in the biblical portrayals of the incarnate Son is to be read back into the intra-Trinitarian divine life. He rather gently critiques and then rejects the "element of 'subordinationism' in [Barth's] doctrine of the Holy Trinity."[19] Torrance follows his reading of Gregory of Nazianzus in rejecting relations of "superiority and inferiority or 'degrees of Deity' in the Trinity" as "quite unacceptable, for to 'subordinate any of the three Divine Persons' is to overthrow the Trinity."[20] Thus "the statement of Jesus 'My Father is greater than I' is to be interpreted not ontologically but soteriologically, or economically... In other words, the subjection of Christ to the Father in his incarnate economy as the suffering and obedient Servant cannot be read back into the eternal hypostatic relations and distinctions subsisting in the Holy Trinity."[21] Paul D. Molnar concludes that "this is not just a patristic insight but a biblically based patristic insight"; thus "there is for Torrance no way that scripture can be read to imply subordinationism within the immanent Trinity."[22]

Returning to Barth, he clearly interprets the subordination of the Son in an eternal sense. He insists that the subordination of the Son somehow

[13] Barth, *Church Dogmatics* II/2, p. 106.   [14] Barth, *Church Dogmatics* IV/1, p. 164.
[15] Barth, *Church Dogmatics* IV/1, p. 164.   [16] Barth, *Church Dogmatics* IV/1, p. 164.
[17] Barth, *Church Dogmatics* IV/1, p. 201.   [18] Barth, *Church Dogmatics* IV/1, p. 202.
[19] Thomas F. Torrance, *Karl Barth: Biblical and Evangelical Theologian* (Edinburgh: T&T Clark, 2001), pp. 131–132.
[20] Thomas F. Torrance, *The Christian Doctrine of God: One Being, Three Persons* (Edinburgh: T&T Clark, 1996), p. 179.
[21] Torrance, *The Christian Doctrine of God*, p. 180.
[22] Paul D. Molnar, *Divine Freedom and the Immanent Trinity: In Dialogue with Karl Barth and Contemporary Theology* (London: T&T Clark, 2002), p. 324.

belongs to the person of the Son *qua* Son in the life of the immanent Trinity. He insists on this point while also resolutely insisting that both modalism (of the classical Sabellian variety) and subordinationism (especially of the Arian and other anti-Nicene varieties) are theologically mistaken and indeed disastrous.

4.3.2 Thomas Aquinas on the Son's Missional Obedience

Thomas Aquinas consistently interprets the Christ of Hebrews through the lens of Niceno-Constantinopolitan and Chalcedonian orthodoxy. He understands the Christology of Hebrews as distinctly "two-natures" Christology, and this clearly informs his interpretation throughout. Contemporary exegetes may criticize Aquinas for reading orthodoxy *back into* the text, but, as Daniel Keating argues, "in most cases" his strategy "casts light on the text and helps to resolve genuine tensions within the letter itself."[23] For not only does the text depict Jesus "as a vulnerable human being who was tempted" and "who was driven to cry out to the Father with tears" while learning obedience through suffering, it also "contains some of the strongest assertions of the eternity and divinity of Christ in the New Testament."[24] In other words, the incarnate Son is fully human without ceasing to be fully divine, and we are to read the witness of Hebrews accordingly.

Turning to his understanding of the Son's "learned obedience," Aquinas is representative of a great deal of the Christian tradition in consideration of the subordination and obedience of the Son. On his view, the missions are to be clearly distinguished from the processions, and obedience and subordination pertain only to the mission of the Son as the incarnate Redeemer. In other words, he will have nothing whatsoever to do with any notion of subordination and obedience that is either eternal or necessary. Explicitly echoing Augustine, he says that

> It is not without reason that Scripture mentions both, that the Son is equal to the Father and the Father is greater than the Son, for the first is said on account of the form of God, and the second is said on account of the form

---

[23] Daniel Keating, "Thomas Aquinas and the Epistle to the Hebrews: 'The Excellence of Christ,'" in Jon C. Laansma and Daniel J. Treier, eds., *Christology, Hermeneutics, and Hebrews: Profiles from the History of Interpretation* (New York: Bloomsbury/T&T Clark, 2012), p. 99.

[24] Keating, "Thomas Aquinas and the Epistle to the Hebrews," p. 99.

of a servant, without any confusion. Now the less is subject to the greater. Therefore in the form of a servant Christ is subject to the Father.[25]

Importantly, it is the *incarnate* Son who is subordinate to the Father. This is the case because it is the *incarnate* Son who has *the form of a servant*. Appealing to his account of the communication of attributes, Aquinas then says that as "we are not to understand that Christ is a creature simply (*simpliciter*) but only in his human nature…so also are we to understand that Christ is subject to the Father not simply (*simipliciter*) but in his human nature."[26] As the editors of the Blackfriars edition express the point:

> It is, then, the divine Word that is subject to the Father – but, it must be added at once, the divine Word precisely and exclusively as subsisting in a human nature. The relation of the divine Word to the Father in the Trinity is free from any trace of subordination; but, having once assumed a human nature, the Son can perform those actions which express subordination.[27]

So Aquinas is strikingly clear that all acceptable senses of subordination must be attributed to the person of the Son *qua-human nature*. Indeed, Aquinas is so certain of this point that he will even insist that the incarnate Son (in his human nature) is subject *to himself*![28] As Thomas Joseph White puts it, "the voluntary human obedience of the Son in temporal history implies a dynamic subordination of his human will to the agency of his transcendent will which he shares with the Father."[29]

Indeed, the unity of the incarnate Son with the Father is of such strength and intensity that Aquinas also insists that Christ enjoys the beatific vision during his earthly career. White explains the point as follows: "Christ as man possessed the immediate, intuitive knowledge of his own deity, the divine life with the Father and the Spirit."[30] This does not mean for Aquinas that Christ had nothing to learn. To the contrary, Aquinas holds that Christ in his human nature surely does have "empiric" or acquired knowledge of

---

[25] Thomas Aquinas, *Summa Theologica* III, q. 20, a.1.

[26] Aquinas, *Summa Theologica* III, q.20, a.1.

[27] Colman E. O'Neill, ed., *The One Mediator*, vol. 50 of *Summa Theologica* (New York: Blackfriars, 1965), pp. 112–113.

[28] Aquinas, *Summa Theologica* III, q.20, a.2.

[29] Thomas Joseph White, O.P., *The Incarnate Lord: A Thomistic Study in Christology* (Washington: Catholic University of America Press, 2015), p. 303.

[30] White, *The Incarnate Lord*, p. 237.

human matters.[31] But it does mean that the incarnate Son is never without direct, filial awareness of his divinity and relationship to his Father.

4.4 Barth's Gambit: A Theological Analysis

As we can see, both Aquinas and Barth affirm that Jesus Christ is subordinate to the Father in some sense. But where Aquinas follows the broadly traditional line of attributing this subordination to the Son *kata sarka* and *forma servi*, to the *incarnate* Word that is, to the Word *qua* humanity, Barth insists that the subordination is proper to the being or divinity of the Triune God.[32] Beyond the observation that these positions are different in some important respects, just what are we to make of their views?

4.4.1 Barth, Consistency, and Monotheism

Barth clearly holds that the subordination of the Son to the Father is somehow internal to the life of the Triune God. "We can say quite calmly," he says, that God "exists as a first and a second, above and below, *a priori* and *a posteriori*."[33] He is well aware that his view will prompt criticism; thus he insists that to "grasp" his point we "have to free ourselves from two unfortunate and very arbitrary ways of thinking."[34] Nonetheless, several puzzles and problems attend Barth's view.

First, it is not hard to see the appearance of inconsistency between what Barth says here and what Barth says elsewhere about the distinction of the divine persons. Barth is well known for his vehement opposition to any doctrine of the Trinity according to which there are multiple divine "centers of consciousness." As he puts it,

---

[31] When I say "Aquinas," I mean the Aquinas of the *ST* (*Summa Theologica*). As Thomas himself notes, by the writing of the *ST* he has changed his mind (from earlier comments on Lombard's *Sentences*). See Aquinas, *Summa Theologica* III. q12. a2.

[32] As Darren Sumner nicely characterizes Barth's position, "Obedience and Subordination in Karl Barth's Trinitarian Theology," in Oliver D. Crisp and Fred Sanders, eds., *Advancing Trinitarian Theology: Explorations in Constructive Dogmatics* (Grand Rapids: Zondervan Academic, 2015), p. 131.

[33] Barth, *Church Dogmatics* IV/1, pp. 201–202.

[34] Barth, *Church Dogmatics* IV/1, p. 202.

By Father, Son, and Spirit we do not mean what is commonly designated to us by the word "persons." This designation was accepted – though not without opposition – on linguistic presuppositions which no longer obtain today. It was never intended to imply – at any rate in the theological tradition – that there are in God three different personalities, three self-existent individuals with their own self-consciousness, cognition, volition, activity, effects, revelation, and name. The one name of the one God is the threefold name of Father, Son, and Holy Spirit. The one "personality" of God, the one active and speaking divine Ego, is Father, Son, and Holy Spirit. Otherwise we should obviously have to speak of three gods.[35]

The notion that there are multiple divine subjects or agents is rejected by Barth as "mythology, for which there can be no place in a right understanding of the doctrine of the Trinity as the doctrine of the three modes of being of the one God ... "[36] Instead, "Christian faith and the Christian confession has one Subject, not three. But he is the one God in self-repetition, in the repetition of his own and equal divine being, and therefore in three different modes of being – which the term 'person' was always explained to mean."[37]

We should note that Barth mixes several distinct claims together. He lumps "three divine personalities" with "three self-existent individuals," and he further conflates both notions with any account of the divine persons according to which they are (or possess) any distinct agency. But it is less than obvious that these come as a kind of package deal that must taken together and then either accepted or rejected accordingly. If there is a relationship of mutual entailment between three "self-existent individuals" and what we might refer to as distinct divine speech-agents, then it is not an *obvious* one. Surely any proponent of orthodox Trinitarian theology would deny that there are three self-existent divine individuals! But to deny this is not to deny that there are three divine speakers or agents, three who know one another.

Questions abound. Is Barth really rejecting the modern psychological definition of person—or is he really assuming it and then insisting that there can only be one such "Ego" within God? Is it really true that an I-Thou relationship within the Trinity would imply multiple deities? Indeed, is not

---

[35] Barth, *Church Dogmatics* IV/1, pp. 204–205.
[36] Barth, *Church Dogmatics* IV/1, p. 65. See also *Church Dogmatics* I/1, pp. 348–368.
[37] Barth, *Church Dogmatics* IV/1, p. 205.

this exactly what the New Testament demands?[38] What does it mean to deny that the divine persons have distinct "activity?" Consider the *opera ad extra*. While Barth is right that the tradition has insisted that these are "always undivided," it is also true that this divine action may be such that it sometimes reaches it terminus on one or another of the divine persons. Thus it is beyond dispute that only the Son became incarnate, for "one of the Trinity suffered in the flesh."[39] Or consider the *opera ad intra*; the generation of the Son is the work of the Father only and not the agency of the Son or Spirit.

If Barth means only that the divine persons are not *self-existent individuals*, then surely he is right. But if he means that they are not distinct in knowledge or agency at all, then it is hard to see how he might be correct about this. At any rate, it is hard to see how his account of intra-Trinitarian subordination is internally consistent with what he says elsewhere about the personhood of God. But pressing beyond the issues of the appearance of inconsistency, however, some critics raise further concerns at this point. For instance, White worries that Barth's doctrine "renders obscure the confession of the unity of the divine will and power in God."[40] For according to classical Trinitarian theology, the Father and Son share exactly one will; on Barth's proposal, on the other hand, the Father always wills that the Son obey and the Son always obeys (albeit in willing agreement). Darren O. Sumner responds on Barth's behalf at this juncture by making three points. First, he says, Barth's account of the subordination of the Son "continues to operate under" his strident critique of any version of "social Trinitarianism."[41] Second, he thinks that Barth "would not be quick to grant the presumption that the act of obedience necessarily entails two willing agents."[42] I cannot see how Sumner's first point does anything but heighten the sense that there is an internal contradiction in Barth's theology, and his second point also fails to provide help. Perhaps it is true that Barth would not have been quick to grant that the problematic conclusion is entailed by his view. But that seems irrelevant to the main point; someone's reluctance to admit that P entails Q is irrelevant to the issue of whether or not P actually

---

[38] See my summary in Jason S. Sexton, ed., *Two Views on the Doctrine of the Trinity* (Grand Rapids: Zondervan Academic, 2014), pp. 117–127.

[39] See Barth himself on this point, *Church Dogmatics* I/1, p. 397.

[40] Thomas Joseph White, O.P., *The Incarnate Lord: A Thomistic Study in Christology* (Washington: Catholic University of America Press, 2015), p. 280.

[41] Sumner, "Obedience and Subordination," p. 140.

[42] Sumner, "Obedience and Subordination," p. 141.

entails Q. Sumner's third rejoinder (to White's critique) is perhaps more promising but surely more perplexing, for he appeals to Barth's "actualistic ontology." According to the "revisionist" interpretation of Barth's "actualism" (especially as defended by Bruce L. McCormack),[43] God elects to be Triune and incarnate and thus is never (at least proleptically) without his humanity. According to this view, the divinity and humanity are in a "mutually conditioning relation" that is eternal.[44] Whether this revisionist interpretation of Barth aids his view or brings it to ruin is a question of intense debate.[45] We need not, however, finally resolve that hotly contested matter to see further worries about Barth's view.

Suppose that the "revisionists" are wrong. In that case, I take it that the correct reading of Barth's view would be

(~R) the will of the eternal Son *qua* Son is eternally and necessarily subordinate to the Father.

Or suppose that the revisionists are right. Then Barth's view would be

(R) the will of the eternal Son *qua humanity* (or, perhaps, *qua the Son's humanity-conditioned deity*) is eternally and necessarily subordinate to the Father.[46]

If (~R) is the right way to take Barth, then we are left to wonder why his view would not qualify as (what he labels) "the worst and most extreme expression of tritheism" and "mythology." Indeed, we are left to wonder why his theology would not be hoist on its own petard. If (R), on the other hand, is the correct reading of Barth, then it seems that its merits are pretty well

---

[43] See especially Bruce L. McCormack, "Grace and Being: The Role of God's Gracious Election i n Karl Barth's Theological Ontology," in John Webster, ed., *The Cambridge Companion to Karl Barth* (Cambridge: Cambridge University Press, 2000), pp. 92–110. Also important is Bruce L. McCormack, " 'With Loud Cries and Tears': The Humanity of the Son in the Epistle to the Hebrews," in Richard Bauckham, Daniel R. Driver, Trevor A. Hart and Nathan MacDonald, eds., *The Epistle to the Hebrews and Christian Theology* (Grand Rapids: William B. Eerdmans Publishing Co., 2009), pp. 37–58.

[44] Sumner, "Obedience and Subordination," pp. 141–142.

[45] George Hunsinger, *Reading Barth with Charity: A Hermeneutical Proposal* (Grand Rapids: Baker Academic, 2015); Paul D. Molnar, *Faith, Freedom, and the Spirit: The Economic Trinity in Barth, Torrance, and Contemporary Theology* (Downers Grove: InterVarsity Academic, 2015); and Michael Dempsey, ed., *Trinity and Election in Contemporary Theology* (Grand Rapids: William B. Eerdmans Publishing Co., 2011). For further discussion, see Chapter 3.

[46] See Sumner, "Obedience and Subordination," pp. 141–142.

camouflaged. For if (R) is right, and if the subordination of the Son belongs to the life of the immanent Trinity, then it seems that we are left with two options. Either the creation of humanity is necessary for God (so that the Son could have a human will with which to condition his divinity) or the Trinity is contingent. Surely the second option would be unpalatable to Barth, so we are left with the first. But does not this option lead straight to panentheism?[47]

4.4.2 Barth and the Threat of Ontological Subordination: The Authority of the Father

A second problem is potentially more serious. Do not Barth's claims about an "above and below" within the Trinity not entail some kind of *ontological* (rather than merely functional or economic) subordinationism? Surely this would be problematic for any Christology that wishes to maintain contact with classical orthodoxy. Barth recognizes the appearance of a problem, and he understands that it would indeed be a serious one. But he denies that this is really a problem for his view. He rejects the assumption that "there is necessarily something unworthy of God and incompatible with His being as God in supposing that there is in God a first and a second, an above and a below, since this includes a gradation, a degradation, and an inferiority in God, which if conceded excludes the *homoousia* of the different modes of the divine being."[48] So while Barth recognizes the appearance of a serious threat to orthodoxy, he refuses to concede that there really is such a problem. At one level he admits that the concern is plausible: "that all sounds very illuminating."[49] But his retort is swift. "Is it not an all too human—and therefore not a genuinely human—way of thinking?"[50] "What is the measure," he wants to know, "by which it measures and judges? Has there really to be something mean in God for Him to be the second, below? Does

---

[47] For analysis of some of these issues, see Chapter 3.

[48] Barth, *Church Dogmatics* IV/1, p. 202. Kevin J. Vanhoozer appears to hold a similar position. After claiming to see "some textual evidence" for eternal submission (in John 5:30; 8:28), he concludes: "suffice it to say that there is nothing necessarily demeaning in suggesting that God the Son is eternally, yet *freely*, obedient to God the Father," *Remythologizing Theology: Divine Action, Passion, and Authorship* (Cambridge: Cambridge University Press, 2010), pp. 255, 256 n59.

[49] Barth, *Church Dogmatics* IV/1, p. 202.   [50] Barth, *Church Dogmatics* IV/1, p. 202.

subordination in God necessarily involve an inferiority, and therefore a deprivation, a lack?"[51] Instead, he asks, "why not rather a particular being in the glory of the one equal Godhead, in whose inner order there is also, in fact, the direction downwards, that has its own dignity? Why should not our way of finding a lesser dignity and significance in what takes the second and subordinate place (the wife to her husband) need to be corrected in light of the *homoousia* of the modes of the divine being?"[52]

Barth's protests notwithstanding, the concerns are serious, and the threat seems real. White worries that Barth's Christology would "make problematic the affirmation of a divine immutable omnipotence present in the incarnate Son."[53] If the Father has authority necessarily and eternally while the Son does not, then it surely seems that they are of different essences. Even Hunsinger says that on Barth's own premises, "obedience is constitutive of the Son's essential deity," and that "obedience belongs to the Son's eternal essence."[54] But if obedience is part of *the Son's* "essential deity" and "belongs to *the Son's* eternal essence" in contradistinction to the Father, then it will be hard to avoid the conclusion that the Son has a different essence. If Barth is right that the Son is obedient "necessarily" and "essentially," then obedience is part of the Son's essence.[55] But if the Father is not obedient "necessarily" and "essentially"—and for Barth the Father most decidedly is *not* obedient at all (much less necessarily and essentially)— then obedience is not part of the Father's essence. Thus the Father and Son are not, *and cannot be, homoousios.* No wonder, then, that even someone as sympathetic to Barth as Molnar admits that Barth "creates a major problem here by introducing hierarchy into the divine being."[56] White concludes that there is "an inevitable discord between [Barth's] affirmation that the eternal,

[51]   Barth, *Church Dogmatics* IV/1, p. 202.
[52]   Barth, *Church Dogmatics* IV/1, p. 202. Barth's appeal to gender and nuptial relations at this point is somewhat puzzling. Exactly what role the appeal to marital relations is to play here is less than obvious, for Barth wants to offer a genuinely theological correction of common notions of husband-wife relations while also drawing upon common relationships between husbands (who, apparently, are authoritative and thus analogous to the Father) and wives (who, apparently, are subordinate and thus analogous to the Son) to support his claim that the Son can be necessarily subordinate to the Father though still equal to him. Moreover, it is not at all clear just how this appeal to gender relations might cohere with his resolute denial of any *vestigium trinitatis*. Molnar asks if Barth himself has not "conceived of the Trinity in an all-too-human way," and he concludes that Barth "has illegitimately read back into the Godhead the order he thinks he found in male-female relations," *Faith, Freedom, and the Spirit*, p. 337.
[53]   White, *The Incarnate Lord*, p. 280.
[54]   Hunsinger, *Reading Barth with Charity*, p. 113.
[55]   Barth, *Church Dogmatics* IV/1, p. 164.
[56]   Molnar, *Faith, Freedom, and the Spirit*, p. 331.

wise, and omnipotent God became human, and [his] affirmation that there is obedience within the very life of God that characterizes the person of the Son as distinct from the Father."[57] More could be said, but it should be obvious that there are deep problems for Barth's view of the obedience and subordination of the Son.[58]

4.4.3   Barth and Hebrews 5

Beyond these general theological concerns—troubling though they are in their own right—we come to the question of how Barth's view relates to the teaching of Hebrews 5. Barth does not offer extended exegesis of this passage, but he does offer some indication of his views.[59] He thinks that the "days of his flesh" refer to his passion and especially to his death.[60] He is certain that the "loud cries and tears" are an "insufficiently noticed" commentary on Gethsemane.[61] He also says that this is a reference to Jesus's cry of dereliction from the cross.[62] And, of course, he is sure that the obedience of the Son is necessary and essential to the Son. This much is obvious. But when we move beyond what Barth says explicitly about this passage and read Hebrews 5 while asking what it means for his general view of Christ's subordination, two main considerations emerge. First, in Hebrews we see that Jesus "*learned*" obedience. On Barth's view, however, obedience and submission are intrinsic to the Son's identity. To be Son is to be "below," the *posterius*, the "Second," the one who "obeys in humility." But if to be the Son is to be obedient, if there is no possibility that the Son is not obedient, then

---

[57] White, *The Incarnate Lord*, p. 280. White suggests that a more "benign" interpretation of Barth is to take this in reference only to the mission of the Son (rather than the procession); he also recognizes that this seems to be at some distance from the most plausible reading of Barth and an even greater distance from the McCormackian "revisionist" account of Barth.

[58] For somewhat more technical treatments of these problems, see, e.g., Thomas H. McCall, *Which Trinity? Whose Monotheism? Philosophical and Systematic Theologians on the Metaphysics of Trinitarian Theology* (Grand Rapids: William B. Eerdmans Publishing Co., 2010), pp. 175–188; Thomas H. McCall and Keith E. Yandell, "On Trinitarian Subordinationism," *Philosophia Christi* (2009), pp. 339–358; Thomas H. McCall, "Gender and the Trinity Once More: A Review Article," *Trinity Journal* (2015), pp. 263–280.

[59] He mentions this passage several times in the *Church Dogmatics* I/1, pp. 386–387; I/2, p. 158; II/2, p. 666; III/2, pp. 327–329, 337, 462; IV/1, pp. 164–165, 193–196; IV/2, pp. 95, 250, 606–607; IV/3, p. 395.

[60] E.g., Barth, *Church Dogmatics* III/2, p. 562.

[61] Barth, *Church Dogmatics* III/2, p. 337; cf. *Church Dogmatics* IV/2, pp. 95, 250.

[62] E.g., Barth, *Church Dogmatics* I/1, p. 386; *Church Dogmatics* I/2, p. 158.

what does it even mean to assert that he *learned* obedience? We do not know, and Barth's Christology gives us little guidance here.[63]

Second, we should remember that he learned obedience *"although"* he was Son. The noun is anarthrous here (as it is in 1:2), and surely this testifies to the quality of his filial relation.[64] When we see this combined with the concessive force of καίπερ, we can see that the force of this statement "is that Jesus is not an ordinary Son, who might be expected to learn through suffering (12:4-11), but the eternal Son."[65] As Luke Timothy Johnson notes, the statement here comes as something of a surprising reversal. We would expect someone to be obedient *because* he is a son, and we indeed are easily tempted to say "because" for καίπερ. But this would be a mistake, he says, because the concessive that is used here actually sets up a *contrast*.[66] Thus William L. Lane concludes that "discussion of the obedience of the Christ is qualified by the affirmation that Jesus is inherently and intrinsically the Son of God, whose essential sonship is a fact wholly apart" from the fact that he learned obedience through suffering.[67] There is no hint here that obedience is constitutive of his Sonship. Hebrews does not lead us to conclude that the filial relationship is based upon that obedience, or even that it entails that obedience. He is obedient *although* he is Son. Accordingly, it is hard to see how Barth's account of the subordination of the Son as necessary and eternal can be consistent with what is stated in Hebrews 5.

4.5 Obedience and the Beatific Vision: Reconsidering Aquinas's View

We have seen that Thomas Aquinas takes a very different view of the subordination and obedience of the Son. The obedience and subordination

---

[63] In the first part of the first volume of the *Dogmatics*, Barth echoes both Hebrews 5 and Philippians 2 in reminding us that the obedience was the obedience of suffering and death on a cross, *Church Dogmatics* I/1, p. 387. By the second part of the first volume, Barth says that "Jesus Christ's obedience consists in the fact that He willed to be and was only this one thing with all its consequences, God in the flesh, the divine bearer of the burden that man as sinner must bear," *Church Dogmatics* I/2, p. 156. He also notes that "the New Testament has nowhere attempted to describe this 'learning,'" p. 158.

[64] Bruce, *Hebrews*, p. 104.

[65] Attridge, *Hebrews*, p. 152. Cf. Craig R. Koester, *Hebrews: A New Translation and Commentary*, The Anchor Bible (New York: Doubleday, 2001).

[66] Luke Timothy Johnson, *Hebrews: A Commentary* (Louisville: Westminster John Knox Press, 2006), p. 147.

[67] Lane, *Hebrews 1–8*, p. 120.

of the Son is to be understood only with reference to the economy of salvation. As such, it pertains only to the mission of the Logos and not to the procession per se. For while the divine missions are, of course, consistent with the divine processions, they are not to be confused or conflated. Nor can we reduce the processions to the missions. The subordination of the Son is for us and our salvation; it is "a dynamic subordination of his human will" to the one divine will that is shared with the Father.[68] Accordingly, Aquinas avoids the problems that are raised by Barth's view. The point here is not that Aquinas merely has different resources than Barth to deal with the problems, rather, the point is that he does not run into these problems at all.

But if Aquinas avoids the problems that come with Barth's view, does his own view not encounter other problems? Here Hebrews 5 is very important, and reflection on it might raise some potential criticisms of Aquinas's view. First, there is a general concern that such Christology would try to import something into this text that is not really present. Aquinas himself appeals to Hebrews 5:8 as an example of Christ's "empiric" or acquired knowledge that he has in virtue of the incarnation.[69] However, Cockerill warns us not to assume too much when reading this text, and especially not to "import the preexistence-humiliation-exaltation schema from Phil 2:6-11 into this passage."[70] He says that the author of Hebrews "certainly assumes the incarnation here, but he says nothing about the preexistent act of obedience by which he became incarnate. God's declaration of sonship and priesthood in vv. 5-6 did not occur in the Son's preexistence but at his exaltation. Verses 7-8 describe the obedient course of his human life. This earthly obedience is integral to both the theological development and pastoral purpose of Hebrews. It is by this obedience that Christ becomes the 'Source' of salvation and thus the one who enables the obedience of his people. His obedience is also their example and encouragement."[71] A canonically informed reading of the text, however, would find what *is* stated here in Hebrews 5 to be entirely consistent with what Paul teaches in Phil 2 (and elsewhere). And, as Cockerill points out, this text actually "assumes the incarnation" while directly addressing "the obedient course of his human life" as "earthly obedience." In sum, one need not read all of

[68] White, *The Incarnate Lord*, p. 303.   [69] Aquinas, *Summa Theologica* III q.9, a.4.
[70] Gareth Lee Cockerill, *The Epistle to the Hebrews*, New International Commentary on the New Testament (Grand Rapids: William B. Eerdmans Publishing Co., 2012), p. 242 n62.
[71] Cockerill, *Hebrews*, p. 242 n62.

Aquinas's Christology *into* the teaching of Hebrews 5 to see that it is consistent with that teaching at this point.

Another potential problem for Aquinas's Christology might come from reflection on the statements that Jesus "offered up prayers and petitions with fervent cries and tears" (5:7) and "learned obedience" (5:8). Is the teaching of Hebrews 5 consistent with Aquinas's steadfast belief in the beatific vision? What could it mean to say that he "learned" obedience (or anything else) if he is omniscient? And what should we make of his "fervent cries and tears" if he really enjoys the beatific vision?

When considering the issue of Christ "learning" obedience, it is hard to see that there is any more of a problem here than there is anywhere else in Aquinas's doctrine of the hypostatic union (and, in particular, his view of the distinction of the natures).[72] He offers an account of the acquisition of knowledge in Christ. Aquinas's doctrine is not, of course, beyond dispute, and his critics (both medieval and modern) are not convinced that his view is finally defensible (his defenders, of course, are convinced that it is). Full consideration of such matters is beyond the scope of the current discussion, but it is hard to see how there might be more of a problem with respect to his learning obedience than there is with him learning anything else. And when we remember that the issue is of learning *obedience*, the message of Hebrews comports nicely with Aquinas's view. As Cockerill notes, the author of Hebrews "is not speaking of a heavenly obedience but of an abandonment to God that occurred when the Son was experiencing all the impairments of a humanity like our earthly humanity."[73]

But what about the "fervent cries and tears" of our Lord? How does this teaching cohere with the conviction that the one who cries out in this way enjoys uninterrupted and untarnished communion with God? In light of this clear teaching in Hebrews, just what are we to make of Aquinas's belief that Christ enjoyed the beatific vision? Two observations are important here. First, we need to see that it seems entirely possible to accept Aquinas's general doctrine of the incarnation (including the metaphysics of the doctrine) without committing ourselves to all the details—and particularly so with respect to his belief in the beatific vision. Many other theologians,

---

[72] For more on Aquinas's metaphysics of the incarnation, see especially Eleonore Stump, *Aquinas* (New York: Routledge, 2003), pp. 407–426; Eleonore Stump, "Aquinas's Metaphysics of the Incarnation," in Stephen T. Davis, Daniel Kendall, SJ, and Gerald O'Collins, SJ, eds., *The Incarnation: An Interdisciplinary Symposium on the Incarnation of the Son of God* (Oxford: Oxford University Press, 2002), pp. 197–218.

[73] Cockerill, *Hebrews*, p. 243.

especially those in the Reformed tradition, take this option by agreeing with a broadly Thomist (or, more minimally, a concretist) account of the metaphysics of the incarnation while also steering clear of the claims about the beatific vision.[74] It seems entirely possible to agree with what he says about the subordination of the Son without also adopting his account of the beatific vision.

Second, it is important not to assume too quickly that Aquinas's doctrine must be inconsistent with this text. Aquinas is, of course, well acquainted with the passage, and he even appeals to it to demonstrate that Christ has acquired knowledge (as well as knowledge that is infused into his human soul). On his "two natures" interpretation of the "learning," Aquinas says that "although Christ knew by simple recognition (*simplici notitia*) what obedience is, he nonetheless learned from the things he suffered."[75] John Calvin is convinced that there is "no doubt" that the loud cries are the prayers from Gethsemane and the cry of dereliction from the cross. He interprets the εὐλαβείας (of v. 7) as terror before the righteous judgment of God (rather than as the reverence that is appropriate to human encounter with God). Jesus is under the curse of God, and he knows it.[76] P. E. Hughes agrees but goes even further, on his interpretation, Jesus fears not only death by execution but also "something other and deeper," and this "other and deeper" fear is truly terrifying. It is nothing short of the "disintegrating experience of separation from God" as Christ is "torn away from his Father."[77] On Aquinas's view, by contrast, Christ's beatific vision gives him the clearest and brightest access to the beauty and goodness of God—the beauty and goodness that the man Jesus Christ shares in the hypostatic union.

If the interpretation of Calvin and Hughes is right, then there indeed seems to be a problem for Aquinas's Christology at this point; it really does look like it would run afoul of the teaching of Hebrews. But is the Calvin-Hughes interpretation correct? There are reasons to doubt that it is. Here are three. First, it is far from obvious that we should interpret the "reverence" or "fear" this way. There are easier and more direct ways to communicate anxiety, dread, or terror; φόβος is at hand and ready for use, but the author of Hebrews does not employ it here. And, as Patrick Gray argues, all uses of

---

[74] E.g., Francis Turretin, *Institutes of Elenctic Theology: Volume Two*, trans. George Musgrave Giger, ed. James T. Dennison, Jr. (Philipsburg, NJ: Presbyterian and Reformed, 1992), p. 354.

[75] Aquinas, *Hebrews*, p. 117.   [76] Calvin, *Hebrews*, pp. 64–65.

[77] Hughes, *Hebrews*, p. 183. I say "goes even further" because Calvin will nonetheless say that "at no time" is the Son "deprived of God's mercy and help," *Hebrews*, p. 64.

εὐλαβείας in the New Testament are "unequivocally positive" and appear in reference to devout and pious worshipers.[78] Certainly it is used positively in Hebrews with reference to Noah (11:7), and overall "there is more than ample precedent for viewing the εὐλαβείας description of Jesus in Heb 5:7 as something other than a picture of cowering fear in the face of death."[79] As Thomas R. Schreiner concludes, "reverence" is a better term than either anxiety or fear.[80] And, importantly, reverence is entirely consistent with the beatific vision. Indeed, how could one have the beatific vision and *not* be reverent? Second, it is far from clear that the cry of dereliction is even in view here. As Ben Witherington III points out, the *multiple* prayers mentioned here in Hebrews do not line up neatly with *the* cry of dereliction.[81] Finally, and much more importantly, to conclude that Christ cries out in terror because he anticipates being "torn apart" from his Father both over-reads the cry of dereliction and is itself inconsistent with the Christian doctrine of God (as I have argued elsewhere).[82] In sum, it is hard to think that there is a significant obstacle to Aquinas's view here in this passage.

But does enjoyment of the beatific vision still somehow damage Christ's soteriological suitability? Is there reason to think that somehow the beatific vision would disqualify the incarnate Son? On Aquinas's view of the incarnation, the human nature of Christ is united with the divine nature, but it is not replaced or overwhelmed by it. The human nature, though unstained by sin, nonetheless relates to the divine as human. Christ is thus able to cry out in solidarity and sympathy with his fellow humans. Moreover, it is precisely *because* his human nature is unsullied by depravity and self-centered sin that he is able to *completely and fully* identify with those to whom he is joined. It is because he is so radically *unselfish* that he is able to "sympathize" so fully as high priest and offer himself so completely for the sins of the world. It is because he is divine as well as human that he is able to be the "Source" of salvation, for no one who is merely human can qualify as Savior who reunites us to God. And it is because he is the one who is human and

[78] Patrick Gray, *Godly Fear: The Epistle to Hebrews and the Greco-Roman Critiques of Superstition* (Atlanta: Society of Biblical Literature, 2003), p. 203.

[79] Gray, *Godly Fear*, p. 203.

[80] Thomas R. Schreiner, *Hebrews*, Biblical Theology for Christian Proclamation (Nashville: B&H Publishing Group, 2015), p. 163.

[81] Ben Witherington III, *Letters and Homilies for Jewish Christians: A Socio-Rhetorical Commentary on Hebrews, James and Jude* (Downers Grove: InterVarsity Academic, 2007), p. 201.

[82] See Thomas H. McCall, *Forsaken: The Trinity and the Cross, and Why It Matters* (Downers Grove: InterVarsity Academic, 2012).

divine—and thus the one who enjoys and is sustained by the beatific vision—that he is able to fully sympathize with us in our weaknesses while also uniting us to God. He is able to be the High Priest, the one who is able to save us from death, because he is both human and divine—and he has the beatific vision precisely because he is the man who is fully divine.

4.6 Conclusion

We have arrived at the point where we can see that while Barth's account of the subordination of the Son both encounters several weighty theological objections and sits awkwardly with the teaching of Hebrews 5:7-10, Aquinas's Christology avoids these problems and coheres well with this passage. While there may be some remaining questions about the overall suitability of some of the more controversial aspects of Thomistic Christology, such questions sit lightly to the central issues at hand. In other words, it is entirely possible to take what Aquinas says about the incarnation more generally and about subordination in particular without committing oneself to what may be more questionable aspects of Aquinas's doctrine.

Even the most casual reader will recognize that my sentiments are with Aquinas rather than Barth on this matter. But we should also see and appreciate the magnificent insights offered by Barth. We should remember that his discussion of the subordination of the Son comes in the context of an extended and insightful discussion of hamartiology. Barth refuses to consider sin apart from a properly Christological center; for Barth it is not "clear how it can be otherwise than that a doctrine of sin which precedes Christology and is independent of it should consciously or unconsciously, directly or indirectly, move in the direction of [idolatry]."[83] Thus he insists upon starting with Christ; in direct opposition to traditional ways of thinking about sin he insists that "in opposition to [such ways] we maintain the simple thesis that only when we know Jesus Christ do we really know that man is the man of sin, what sin is, and what it means for us."[84] What we do learn about sin in light of Christ is not at all flattering:

---

[83] Barth, *Church Dogmatics* IV/1, p. 365.   [84] Barth, *Church Dogmatics* IV/1, p. 389.

Man wants only to judge. He thinks he sits on a high throne, but in reality he sits only on a child's stool, blowing his little trumpet, cracking his little whip, pointing with frightful seriousness his little finger, while all the time nothing happens that really matters. He can only play the judge. He is only a dilettante, a blunderer, in his attempt to distinguish between good and evil, right and wrong, acting as though he really had the capacity to do it. He can only pretend to himself and others..."[85]

This is because sin, "in its totality is pride."[86] It is pride and "sloth" (disobedience as a manifestation of unbelief), and it takes many forms: stupidity, inhumanity, dissipation, inordinate care about trivialities.[87] And while pride manifests itself as trying to be like God, it only does so by trying to take the place of a "god" that does not exist. The sad error is that this idolatry only yields a "god" who is "self-centered."[88] But in direct and starkest contrast to such sin, in God incarnate we see not a pitiful and terrifying caricature of God but the God truly revealed in Jesus Christ. And in Christ we see that

> God is for himself, but he is not only for himself. He is in a supreme self-hood, but not a self-contained self-hood, not in a mere divinity...God is *a se* and *per se*, but as the love which is grounded in itself from all eternity. Because he is the triune God, who from the first loved us as the Father in the Son and turned to us by the Spirit, he is God *pro nobis*...God is not egoistic in this revelation and defense of his honor and glory, nor is he concerned about the satisfaction of his needs. As God he does not need...[89]

I take these to be marvelous insights from Barth. Barth is wrong to designate this humility and condescension as somehow unique to *the Son's deity*; the better way is to see this as Christ's revelation of the self-giving love of *the Triune God*. Frankly, his view needs correction: it is not merely *the Son* who is capable of condescension, humility, and self-sacrifice. It is *the Triune God* who is revealed by Jesus Christ as the God who condescends in self-giving love in the incarnation of the Son. Such correction is possible, and in fact it

---

[85] Barth, *Church Dogmatics* IV/1, p. 446.
[86] Barth, *Church Dogmatics* IV/1, p. 414. He also admits that "pride" is a "very feeble word to describe" the human condition; "the correct word is perhaps megalomania," p. 437.
[87] Barth, *Church Dogmatics* IV/2, pp. 404–405.
[88] Barth, *Church Dogmatics* IV/1, p. 422.
[89] Barth, *Church Dogmatics* IV/1, pp. 422, 452.

seems to cohere closely to Barth's own methodological commitments. Jesus Christ is revelatory *of God*, after all. Properly corrected, this powerful truth is one that is consistent with Aquinas's overall Christology. But it is one that finds particularly forceful articulation from Barth. Hopefully, we can learn from both theologians. Hopefully, they will help us to read Hebrews better. And hopefully—by God's grace—we can better know God as Father and walk in holy obedience to him.

5

The Communion of the Son with the Father

5.1 Introduction

In Jesus's famous Johannine "high priestly" prayer, he prays for himself (as "the Son"); specifically he prays that he will be glorified "with the glory I had with you before the world began" (John 17:5). He follows this with prayer for his disciples, and he asks his Father to provide them with strength and sanctity (17:13-19). Further, he prays for those who will believe in him in the future, and he offers prayer for their unity. Strikingly, he prays that the unity of those who know him and who know the Father through him will mirror the unity between Father and Son (17:21-23). He prays that they will know the love of the Father for the Son, and then he adds this striking claim: the love of the Father for the Son is the love given "before the foundation of the world" (John 17:24).

But some influential systematic and philosophical theologians deny that there is any love given and received among the persons of the Trinity. For instance, the prominent analytic theologian Keith Ward says that "to speak of love between the divine persons is virtually vacuous."[1] He denies that there is intra-Trinitarian love in God's own life: "there is no mutual love between Father and Son."[2] Thus he insists that "we should not think of Father and Son apart from creation as exhibiting mutual, relational, and self-giving love."[3] Ward says instead that "self-giving love" exists only "between God and beings other than God."[4] Similarly, Karl Rahner flat-out denies that there is mutual love between the persons of the Trinity; he says that there is "properly no mutual love between the Father and the Son."[5] His rationale for

[1] Keith Ward, "Reimagining the Trinity: On Not Three Gods," *Philosophia Christi* 18:2 (2016), p. 285.
[2] Keith Ward, *Christ and the Cosmos: A Reformulation of Trinitarian Doctrine* (Cambridge: Cambridge University Press, 2015), p. 242.
[3] Ward, *Christ and the Cosmos*, p. 118.   [4] Ward, *Christ and the Cosmos*, p. 231.
[5] Karl Rahner, *The Trinity* (New York: Crossroad, 1997), p. 106.

Analytic Christology and the Theological Interpretation of the New Testament. Thomas H. McCall,
Oxford University Press (2021). © Thomas H. McCall. DOI: 10.1093/oso/9780198857495.003.0006

such denials is not hard to see: mutual love "would presuppose two acts" and thus would be polytheism.[6] Similarly, in his stimulating book entitled *The Model of Love*, the philosophical theologian Vincent Brummer considers the view that "God does not need persons beyond himself in order to be a God of love, for the three persons of the Trinity eternally love each other."[7] Brummer's verdict is swift and decisive: "this view of the Trinity is unsatisfactory for both religious and theological reasons."[8] It is deficient religiously because "a God who does not need to participate in loving fellowship with us is unable to secure our self-esteem and give body to our sense of identity."[9] And it is theologically faulty because this doctrine "cannot do justice to the unity between the persons of the Trinity."[10] Thomas Jay Oord echoes Ward on this point; he claims that "social" views of the Trinity "smack of tritheism" and insists that God has "no divine relations."[11] He is certain that God "has one will, one locus of freedom, one mind, and no internal relations."[12] Working from a very different set of theological commitments, Katherine Sonderegger denies that there is mutual love within the Trinity. For while love indeed is the essence of God, it is ultimately an *object-less* love that thus is not inherently or necessarily relational and that has no object (personal or otherwise). Rejecting both the long-standing Christian tradition (and even disagreeing with Karl Barth) while also rejecting the essential God-world relationality of process theism, she resolutely denies that love is shared between the persons of the Trinity.[13]

These denials are often associated with a critique and rejection of "Social Trinitarianism." If "Social Trinitarianism" (ST) is false—and many theologians are certain that it is—then it must be the case that love is not "internal" to God. On the other hand, other theologians are convinced that "Social Trinitarianism" must be true simply because there indeed *is* love within the Trinity. One side seems to reason along these lines:

---

[6] Rahner, *The Trinity*, p. 106.

[7] Vincent Brummer, *The Model of Love: A Study in Philosophical Theology* (Cambridge: Cambridge University Press, 1993), p. 238.

[8] Brummer, *The Model of Love*, p. 238.   [9] Brummer, *The Model of Love*, p. 238.

[10] Brummer, *The Model of Love*, p. 238.

[11] Thomas Jay Oord, "Can God Be Essentially Loving without Being Essentially Social? An Affirmation of and Alternative for Keith Ward," *Philosophica Christi* 18:2 (2016), p. 356.

[12] Oord, "Can God Be Essentially Loving," p. 353.

[13] E.g., Katherine Sonderegger, *Systematic Theology, Volume One: The Doctrine of God* (Minneapolis: Fortress Press, 2015), pp. 469–490.

(1) If there is love within the (immanent) Trinity, then "Social Trinitarianism" is true;

(2) "Social Trinitarianism" is false;

(3) Therefore, there is no love within the (immanent) Trinity.

The other side appears to think that:

(1) If there is love within the (immanent) Trinity, then "Social Trinitarianism" is true;

(2*) There is love within the (immanent) Trinity;

(3*) Therefore, "Social Trinitarianism" must be true.

This seems to be a classic case of "one theologian's *modus ponens* is another theologian's *modus tollens*." But what are we to make of all this? Is there a clear "winner" in this debate? And, more importantly, how *should* we think about the relationship between the Father and the Son—especially in light of the New Testament witness and particularly in light of the depictions available in John's portrayal of this relationship?

In this chapter, I shall explore so of these matters. I shall do so in close conversation with Ward's emphatically *non-Social Trinitarian* proposal. It is hard to make much progress unless and until we have a reasonably clear sense of what it is that we are talking about, and, since there is a lot of confusion about the meaning of terms like "Social Trinitarianism," in this chapter I first survey some prominent conceptions and common usages of the terms "Social Trinity" and "Social Trinitarianism." Following these ground-clearing exercises, I offer a theological analysis of Ward's non- and anti-ST proposal. Finally, I turn to a consideration of how theological exegesis of the New Testament (and particularly Johannine theology) might inform the current debate.

5.2 The Furor Over Social Trinitarianism: Toward Clarity

Not long ago, "Social Trinitarianism" seemed to be not only the present but also the future of Trinitarian theology. It was central to many discussions of the doctrine of God. Thomas R. Thompson is representative of many when he refers not only to the "doctrinal renaissance" but also the "ethical relevance" and "social redolence" of the doctrine of the Trinity, and he clearly sees this important theological work as deeply and inherently "social" in orientation.[14] The element of "renaissance" or "retrieval" was pronounced, and there was much effort to "recover" the patristic and especially "Eastern" or "Greek" doctrine of the Trinity. And the "ethical relevance" and "social redolence" aspects also generated a great deal of enthusiasm and excitement as great effort was expended in attempts to "apply" the doctrine of the Trinity to a wide range of ethical dilemmas and to further use it as a kind of blueprint for ecclesial and indeed political life. During this "renaissance," however, at many points the notion of ST was not closely defined, and this lack of clarity continues to hamper some of the defenders and proponents of it.

Recent work on the doctrine has seen a very sharp and sustained backlash against ST. The effort to recover an authentically "Eastern" or "Greek" doctrine that differs drastically from "Western" or "Latin" or "Augustinian" accounts is now widely criticized and even belittled by historical theologians. Meanwhile, the search for direct application of the doctrine to socio-political and ethical issues has come under heavy fire; serious methodological weaknesses have been exposed, and worries of projection are now common.[15] In some circles, we seem to have reached a point where the "ST" label can now be used as a term of abuse or derision, or even as a way to dismiss a theological proposal—if some theological proposal X can be identified as "ST," then it does not so much as deserve serious consideration. Indeed, for some of the critics, even to take social accounts of the doctrine seriously is a mistake (as if criticizing the doctrine with genuine respect might sully one's reputation). Unfortunately, however, again there is not a great deal of clarity regarding the use of the term. As Michael Rea and I have pointed out, "Neither the defenders of nor the detractors from Social Trinitarianism have been especially clear about the core tenets of their view."[16]

Richard Bauckham highlights the following elements as "common" to "social" doctrines of the Trinity. First, and "unlike much of the tradition," Social Trinitarians "do not give priority to the one divine substance over the three Persons in God. The three Persons are irreducible."[17] Second, Social

---

[14] Thomas R. Thompson, "Trinitarianism Today: Doctrinal Renaissance, Ethical Relevance, Social Redolence," *Calvin Theological Journal* 32:1 (1997), pp. 9–42.

[15] E.g., Karen Kilby, "Perichoresis and Projection: Problems with Social Doctrines of the Trinity," *New Blackfriars* 81 (2000), pp. 432–445.

[16] Thomas H. McCall and Michael C. Rea, "Introduction," in Thomas H. McCall and Michael C. Rea, eds., *Philosophical and Theological Essays on the Trinity* (Oxford: Oxford University Press, 2009), p. 2.

[17] Richard Bauckham, *Gospel of Glory: Major Themes in Johannine Theology* (Grand Rapids: Baker Academic, 2015), p. 37.

Trinitarians are opposed to psychological analogies and "understand the three Persons to be acting and relating subjects, not the three modes of being of a single personal subject."[18] Third, Social Trinitarians "use the concept of perichoresis (or coinherence or mutual indwelling) to point to a kind of relationship among the three Persons that actually constitutes their unity."[19] And, lastly, they "see a correspondence between the relations within the Trinity and the kind of human relationships, whether in ecclesial or political society, that reflect the trinitarian sociality of God."[20] This is helpful, but let us seek further clarity.

5.2.1 Social Trinitarianism as Socio-Political Advocacy

Sometimes the term "Social Trinitarianism" is used primarily (or perhaps even exclusively) for efforts to "apply" the doctrine of the Trinity in various ecclesial, social, and political ways. If we were to take this as a kind of definition, we would have something like:

(P-ST) Social Trinitarianism = df. *Christian theology that seeks to draw socio-political and ethical implications from the doctrine of the Trinity.*

The past few decades have seen an astoundingly wide range of efforts at "application." Many of these efforts are mutually exclusive, and many of them have been judged to be utterly lacking in argumentative rigor. Karen Kilby has raised serious worries about "projection"; her concern is that we take some favored social program or political ambition and then try to buttress it with "theological support" from the doctrine of the Trinity.[21] Kilby argues that this threatens to make theology only a tool of various (and sometimes competing) socio-political agendas—and thus exemplifies Feuerbach's criticisms of religious belief. The backlash against such approaches has been very strong indeed; thus Stephen R. Holmes goes so far as to say that "the doctrine of the Trinity is necessarily and precisely useless, and that point must never be surrendered."[22] His point is that

---

[18] Bauckham, *Gospel of Glory*, p. 37.
[19] Bauckham, *Gospel of Glory*, p. 37. Bauckham says that this point is "crucial."
[20] Bauckham, *Gospel of Glory*, p. 37.
[21] Kilby, "Perichoresis and Projection," pp. 432–445.
[22] Stephen R. Holmes, "Classical Trinity: Evangelical Perspective," in Jason Sexton, ed., *Two Views on the Doctrine of the Trinity* (Grand Rapids: Zondervan Academic, 2014), p. 47.

knowledge of God is the highest end in itself—the doctrine has no "instrumental use" and "serves no end."[23]

Such criticisms of the efforts at "application" are interesting and sometimes strike me as being very insightful, but this seems misguided as a definition of the term. Fundamentally, this is an account of the *use* of a doctrine rather than an account of the contents of the doctrine itself. Additionally, a wide range of doctrinal proposals can be (and indeed have been) pressed into service for various agendas on a bewilderingly broad range of ethical issues; even Kilby seeks to explore the "dimensions in which an apophatic trinitarianism has potential political significance"—despite the facts that she is both sharply critical of ST and deeply sympathetic to Karl Rahner's theology in her own constructive work![24] So this simply doesn't seem like a helpful employment of the term, and at any rate offers very little of substance with respect to a definition.

5.2.2 "Social Trinitarianism" as "Eastern" (vs. "Western") Theology

Another fairly common use of the term tends to associate it with "Eastern" or "Greek" patristic theology. Accordingly, we might summarize this as something like:

(H-ST) Social Trinitarianism = df. *the doctrine of the Trinity that was held by the major pro-Nicene Greek-speaking theologians of the fourth century (especially Gregory of Nyssa, Gregory of Nazianzus, and Basil of Caesarea), particularly where that doctrine is distinct from the "Latin" or "Western" theology (especially as exemplified by Augustine, Anselm, and Aquinas).*

Where the previous approach employs a more functional usage, this one opts for a more historical account. Of course it is only formal at this level of abstraction, and much work would have to be done to spell out just what it is that the major pro-Nicene theologians believed. Before we even get to such work, however, we run into problems. Unfortunately, however, this

[23] Holmes, "Classical Trinity," pp. 47, 48.
[24] Karen Kilby, "The Trinity and Politics: An Apophatic Approach," in Oliver D. Crisp and Fred Sanders, eds., *Advancing Trinitarian Theology: Explorations in Constructive Dogmatics* (Grand Rapids: Zondervan Academic, 2014), p. 86.

approach does not have much going for it, for there are problems at several levels. First, recent historical work has helped us to see that there are serious differences between important elements of the theology of the major pro-Nicene Greek-speaking theologians of the fourth century, on one hand, and, on the other hand, the theologies of leading proponents of ST in the twentieth and twenty-first centuries. In other words, Gregory of Nyssa and Jürgen Moltmann hold very different views on important matters; we need look no further than the doctrine of divine simplicity to see this. So this historically grounded definition just won't work well to capture the essence of contemporary ST; it doesn't work well *descriptively*. Moreover, and more importantly, this same work in historical theology helps us see that it is a mistake to simplistically pit "Eastern" or "Greek" theology against "Western" or "Latin" theology. It simply isn't the case that "the East" somehow "starts" with "threeness" or emphasizes personhood and "rela-tionality" rather than unity and simplicity while "the West" "starts" with "oneness" and emphasizes simplicity or oneness rather than personhood and relationality. The old clichés have fallen on hard times, for the Cappadocians also believe in divine simplicity (among other doctrines sometimes said to be "Western" or "Latin").[25] I don't deny that there are real differences between Latin and Greek theology, nor do I mean to suggest that such differences are unimportant. The point is rather that the differ-ences are not what the common "Social Trinity" narrative has made them out to be. The upshot of this is that the historical definition doesn't seem any more helpful *prescriptively* than it is useful *descriptively*.

5.2.3 Social Trinitarianism as Theology that Employs the "Social Analogy"

Perhaps the foregoing historical account won't work as a definition but gets us closer to one that can work. Our next proposal is closely related to the previous one. The use of the so-called "social analogy" is well known. Famously, Gregory of Nyssa puts it to work in his "On Not Three Gods." There is a sense in which the God who is Father, Son, and Spirit is analogous to "Peter,

---

[25] For discussion, see, e.g., Andrew Radde-Gallwitz, *Basil of Caesarea, Gregory of Nyssa, and the Transformation of Divine Simplicity* (Oxford: Oxford University Press, 2009); Thomas H. McCall, "Trinity Doctrine, Plain and Simple," in Oliver D. Crisp and Fred Sanders, eds., *Advancing Trinitarian Theology: Explorations in Constructive Dogmatics* (Grand Rapids: Zondervan Academic, 2014), pp. 42–59.

James, and John."[26] Somewhat less famously (if somewhat more ingeniously), Gregory of Nazianzus prefers "Adam, Eve, and Seth" (for here we have one who is unbegotten, one who is begotten, and one who proceeds without being begotten).[27] Accordingly, we might try to define Social Trinitarianism as

(A-ST) Social Trinitarianism = df. *Trinitarian theology that makes positive use of the social analogy; God is relevantly and importantly like three human persons.*

I think that this proposal holds more promise than the others. But it still won't do enough to offer much help by way of definition. First, we should note that it is less than ideal *descriptively* simply because some contemporary proponents of ST do not make use of the social analogy. Some do; Cornelius Plantinga, Jr., for instance, puts it to work in his constructive proposals.[28] But Plantinga does not lean on it hard, and it seems to me that he could make the substantive claims without it. Overall, this account alone does not do much descriptively.

Second, it isn't clear that it will suffice as a satisfactorily substantive *prescriptive* account. For mere use of the analogy doesn't say much; it simply doesn't tell us much at all about the content of the doctrine. The recognition of the important areas of discontinuity and disanalogy are very important here. It is worth noting that the Cappadocians are very quick indeed to point out these areas of discontinuity and to insist on the limits of theological language; we should also note that some contemporary proponents of ST are not nearly so flat-footed as their critics sometimes make them out to be. The analogy itself does not determine the content of the doctrinal claims, and the disclaimers that accompany the analogy are very important.

5.2.4 Social Trinitarianism as Theology that Makes Use of the "Modern Notion" of Person

The foregoing possibilities correspond largely to the positive usage of self-avowed "Social Trinitarians." But another possibility may be more

[26] Gregory of Nyssa, "On Not Three Gods," *NPNF* V, p. 335.
[27] Gregory of Nazianzus, "The Fourth Theological Oration: On the Son," p. 317; and "The Fifth Theological Oration: On the Holy Spirit," *NPNF* VII, p. 322.
[28] Cornelius Plantinga, Jr., "The Threeness/Oneness Problem and the Trinity," *Calvin Theological Journal* 23:1 (1988), pp. 37–53.

commonly associated with the criticisms of it. This is the linkage of the term to distinctly "modern notions" of "personhood." Typical here is the reference to the divine persons as "distinct centers of consciousness" or autonomous individuals, and sometimes ST is charged with importing "Cartesian," "Lockean," or "late Romantic" notions of personhood into the doctrine of the Trinity.[29] Thus we might opt for something like:

(M-ST) Social Trinitarianism = df. *Trinitarian theology that makes positive use of modern (as opposed to traditional) concepts of personhood.*

The critics of ST are correct to point out that different meanings develop for key theological terms over time, and they helpfully caution us against reading "modern notions" into traditional doctrine. But this won't work all that well as an account of what ST *is*. I mention several reasons to think this. First, this won't work well *descriptively*. For in point of fact not all proponents of ST employ modern or contemporary notions of "person" (at least not obviously, and at least not intentionally), and some theologians who are often taken to be defenders of ST actually try to use their doctrines of the Trinity to *criticize and correct* modern notions of personhood.[30] On the other hand, some of the most ferocious *critics* of ST make explicit use of distinctly modern accounts in their own constructive alternative accounts. Brian Leftow is a particularly forceful critic of ST, but he appeals to what he calls "Locke-persons" in his articulation and defense of "Latin Trinitarianism."[31] So at the descriptive level, it isn't at all obvious that commitment to some modern notion of personhood is either necessary or sufficient.

Second, this won't work all that well *prescriptively*, for it isn't an entirely simple matter to so easily oppose "modern" notions to "the traditional" concept. Just as there isn't a single thing called "the modern view," neither is there a single thing called "the traditional perspective." To the contrary, there are multiple accounts of personhood within the tradition. Thomas Aquinas opts for what is basically a Boethian notion of person as "individual substance of a rational nature" (*persona est individua substantia rationalis naturae*).[32]

[29] E.g. Stephen R. Holmes, "Response to Thomas H. McCall," in Jason Sexton, ed., *Two Views on the Doctrine of the Trinity* (Grand Rapids: Zondervan Academic, 2014), p. 143.

[30] E.g., Colin E. Gunton, *The Promise of Trinitarian Theology* (Edinburgh: T&T Clark, 1991).

[31] E.g., Brian Leftow, "Modes Without Modalism," in Peter van Inwagen and Dean Zimmerman, eds., *Persons, Human and Divine* (Oxford: Oxford University Press, 2007), pp. 357–375.

[32] E.g., Thomas Aquinas, *Summa Theologica*. Complete English Edition in Five Volumes, translated by the Fathers of the English Dominican Province (New York: Benzinger Bros., 1948), Ia QQ29.1.

Meanwhile, Richard of St. Victor is well aware of Boethius's definition but is not at all hesitant to disagree with it. Famously, he holds that a divine person is an "incommunicable existence of a divine nature" (*persona divina est divinae naturae incommunicabilis existentia*).[33]

Before moving forward, I think that it is important to note the tendency to exaggerate the differences between "*the* tradition" and "modern" notions. While it certainly is the case that we should be wary of the a-historicizing temptations to flatten out important differences or ignore crucial changes and developments, we should also be vigilant not to over-emphasize the differences or to assume that any change is departure rather than development. Indeed, some excellent historical theologians are also helping us not over-react. For instance, Khaled Anatolios makes some important points while commenting on the theology of Athanasius:

> It has become fashionable to deny that early Christian theology conceived of divine "personhood" in terms anywhere resembling our contemporary understanding of this notion. Be that as it may, we should not overlook the ways in which a theology like Athanasius's, in its careful adherence to the narrative biblical patterns of identifying Father, Son, and Spirit, finds itself depicting the relation between Father and Son in terms that intersect with some aspects of our modern notion of personhood. Certainly, to be a center of conscious intentionality is integral to our modern notion of personhood, and the interactions of subjects so that they become mutual subjects and objects of each other's intentionality and affirmation is integral to our modern conception of intersubjectivity. But the attribution of conscious intentionality to the divine relations is precisely the issue at point in this passage, not because Athanasius has a presciently modern conception of divine or human personhood but simply because he is beholden to the patterns of biblical narrative and symbol.[34]

Anatolios says further that while

> Gregory clarifies elsewhere that there is one movement of will that encompasses the divine being, he is equally clear . . . that this one movement is

---

[33] Richard of St. Victor, *De Trinitate* IV.xxii; *PL* 196 945C. This is in deliberate contradistinction to the definition of Boethius, e.g., *De Trinitate* IV.xxi; *PL* 196 945A.

[34] Khaled Anatolios, *Retrieving Nicaea: The Development and Meaning of Trinitarian Doctrine* (Grand Rapids: Baker Academic, 2011), p. 153. Anatolios's reference to Athanasius is to *Contra Ar.* 3.66.

appropriated by all three *hyposaseis* such that each becomes the subject of the divine will, agency, and power. This might not amount to "modern conceptions of personhood," but neither does it utterly exclude some of these conceptions.[35]

Similarly, and concerning medieval theology, Gilles Emery offers a very helpful word of caution here: "we need not contrast Thomas's metaphysical attitude to the topic with one which stresses the 'psychological' elements of the person (such as life of the mind: knowledge, freedom, action, and openness to another), because these elements are integrated into his own approach."[36] We need to understand the difference between mere repetition and consistency. After all, mere repetition may not even make the same propositional claims in evolving semantic domains and changing intellectual contexts. We also need to understand that not all change equals or entails a rejection or departure. There is such a thing as development of doctrine.

5.2.5 Social Trinitarianism and Intra-Trinitarian Love

ST might be thought of as any doctrine of the Trinity according to which the divine persons love one another. This is, to be sure, very often a strong emphasis of theologians who rally beneath the banner of ST. For example, Plantinga refers to the Holy Trinity as

> a divine, transcendent society or community of three fully personal and fully divine entities: the Father, the Son, and the Holy Spirit or Paraclete. These three are wonderfully united by their common divinity, that is, by the possession of each of the whole generic divine essence...the persons are also unified by their joint redemptive purpose, revelation, and work. Their knowledge and love are directed not only to their creatures, but also primordially and archetypally to each other. The Father loves the Son and the Son loves the Father...the Trinity is thus a zestful community of divine light, love, joy, mutuality, and verve.[37]

---

[35] Anatolios, *Retrieving Nicaea*, pp. 219–220.

[36] Gilles Emery, *The Trinitarian Theology of St Thomas Aquinas* (Oxford: Oxford University Press, 2007), p. 106.

[37] Cornelius Plantinga, Jr., "Social Trinity and Tritheism," in Ronald J. Feenstra and Cornelius Plantinga, Jr., eds., *Trinity, Incarnation, and Atonement: Philosophical and Theological Essays* (Notre Dame: University of Notre Dame Press, 1989), pp. 27–28.

If we work from this position toward a definition of ST, we might get something along the lines of:

> (L-ST) Social Trinitarianism = df. *any doctrine of the Trinity according to which the Father, Son, and Holy Spirit love one another within the intratrinitarian divine life (the "immanent Trinity").*

This approach has the advantage of cohering well with a—perhaps *the*—major emphasis of avowed proponents of ST. But as it stands it is too vague to be of much help as a definition. We shall return to this in due course.

5.2.6 Social Trinitarianism and Distinct Agency

Alternatively, some may think of ST as any theory according to which the divine persons are distinct agents. This is, after all, the way that it is sometimes characterized by its critics. We might think of ST as something like:

> (D-ST) Social Trinitarianism = df. *any doctrine of the Trinity according to which the divine persons are distinct in agency.*

Things get complicated here. It is, of course, a commonplace in historic Christian orthodoxy that the divine actions of God that are "outside" of God are always unified and never divided: *opera ad extra sunt omnia indivisa.* But while it is true that this is catholic teaching, it is not the case that this should be understood in such a way that would rule out any distinction of agency. After all, "undivided" neither equals nor entails "indistinct." It has not, historically, been taken to eliminate any distinction; for all mainstream patristic and medieval theologians, it is true that only the Son becomes incarnate, only the Spirit comes at Pentecost, etc. As even Lewis Ayres (who is no friend of ST) says in commenting on patristic interpretation of Rom 8, it seems as though "there are three actors, each of whom plays a part in bringing the Christian to new life, often in overlapping ways."[38] Whatever

---

[38] Lewis Ayres, " 'As We Are One:' Thinking into the Mystery," in Oliver D. Crisp and Fred Sanders, eds., *Advancing Trinitarian Theology: Explorations in Constructive Dogmatics* (Grand Rapids: Zondervan Academic, 2014), p. 99. Ayres further cautions against the presumption that ST is necessarily "*opposed to* a classical perspective," p. 103 n9 (emphasis original).

exactly the claim that the *opera ad extra* are *indivisa* means, it certainly does not mean anything that is inconsistent with the bedrock claim that only the Son was incarnate and suffered the passion. On pain of patripassianism, it cannot mean anything less. And when we come to the *opera ad intra*, however, matters are even more starkly different. For only the Father generates the Son. So, minimally, there is a prima facie case to be made that any orthodox Christian should not hesitate to affirm that the agency of the divine persons is distinct in some important sense(s).

5.2.7 "Real" Social Trinitarianism

To this point I've surveyed common uses of the term "Social Trinitarianism," and I have explored how these might function if we try to understand them referentially. I have noted challenges for all such uses, I have pointed out that none of them offer much along the lines of a promising way forward, and I have suggested that they may only deepen the confusion that surrounds the use of the term. Surely those who criticize and reject social doctrines of the Trinity—even those who do so with considerable snide and impressive snark—should wish to be clear about just it is that they are against.

In the past, I (along with Michael C. Rea) have suggested that we think about ST rather differently. More precisely, ST can be understood as the conjunction of:

(R-ST1) The Father, Son, and Holy Spirit are "of one essence," but are not numerically the same substance. Rather, the divine persons are consubstantial only in the sense that they share the divine nature in common. Furthermore, this sharing of a common nature can be understood in a fairly straightforward sense via the "social analogy" in which Peter, James, and John share human nature;

(R-ST2) Properly understood, the central claim of monotheism that there is but one God is to understood as the claim that there is one divine nature—not as the claim that there is exactly one divine substance;

and (R-ST3) The divine persons must each be in full possession of the divine nature and in some particular relation R to one another for Trinitarianism to count as monotheism (where the usual candidates for R are being members of the same kind, the only members of the divine family, the only members of a necessarily existent community, enjoying perfect love and harmony of will, and being necessarily interdependent).[39]

5.2.8 Conclusion

So where does this leave us? We should be in a position to see that several of these meanings are not particularly helpful. Some are concerned with issues that are interesting but rather peripheral. I am convinced that the ST label is best reserved for what I here refer to *real* ST (R-ST). But I am, however, also aware that not everyone sees matters as I do and that other uses continue to remain in currency. So while I think it would be best if we were to use the "ST" label only for "R-ST," if we are not going to do that, then we can at least be clear about how we *are* using it. And, for our purposes, what I have referred to as (L-ST) and (D-ST) remain of keen interest, for the depiction of the Father-Son relationship offered in Johannine theology is directly relevant to them.

5.3 An Anti-Social Proposal Analyzed

5.3.1 Ward's Trinitarian Doctrine

Keith Ward has written a fascinating, bold, and powerful exercise in "analytical theology."[40] In contrast to much Trinitarian theology, he utterly rejects any notion that the Trinity is a "society of three subjects of consciousness" (257), and with this rejection he dispenses with the idea of mutual love shared between the divine persons within the life of the immanent Trinity (e.g., x, 117–118, 186). Ward insists that "what Christians claim to know of God as Trinity is dependent upon a divine revelation in the person of Jesus and depends upon the actuality of that person in human history" (91). On this I largely agree with Ward.[41] To be more specific, what Christians can know about God as Trinity is dependent on a divine

---

[39] See McCall and Rea, "Introduction," p. 3.

[40] Keith Ward, *Christ and the Cosmos: A Reformulation of Trinitarian Doctrine* (Cambridge: Cambridge University Press, 2015), p. xv. Subsequent references will hereafter be included parenthetically in the text.

[41] I think that arguments from "perfect being theology" to the doctrine of the Trinity (such as those defended by Richard of St. Victor or Richard Swinburne) demonstrate at most that there must be more than one divine person who relates to the other(s) in mutual love, but such arguments do not get us to the conclusion that there are exactly three such persons.

revelation of Jesus Christ *as the incarnate Son of God*. Ward, I take it, would agree with me about this specification. But just what does this mean? What do we learn of God as Trinity from the incarnate Son? And what are we to make of the incarnation itself? Here, as we shall see, Ward's characteristic clarity starts to fade, and basis for agreement becomes more elusive.

Jesus Christ is central to Ward's discussion of the Synoptic Gospels. He recognizes that Jesus is "worshiped as Lord in the early churches" ("and yet there are not two Gods") even as he is completely human (47). He says that

> Jesus is a man sent and appointed by God to have supreme authority and to rule over other humans in the coming Kingdom, where he will sit at the right hand of God in glory and power. He is the Messiah, the liberator and King, and the Lord of all people, who are to be called his disciples. Such a person is in some sense both human and divine.   (48)

At the same time, however, there are "complications" as well as "limitations" that are related to the humanity and death of Jesus. "So one cannot simply place Jesus, a limited and suffering and dying person, alongside the creator God as identical in every respect" (48). Turning to his consideration of the Fourth Gospel, he rejects "two minds Christology" and instead posits "only one personal 'subject' in Jesus; but it is not the Word, which is not a distinct subject of consciousness and will at all" (56–57). What we have in the Johannine depiction of Jesus, then, is this: "there is only the human subject in Jesus, but that subject perfectly expresses the divine Ideal or self-communicative expression of God" (57). So Jesus is "a real human subject" who is "conformed wholly to the eternal divine Ideal" (57). As Ward explains further, "the Word, on this model, is an eternal possibility made actual, first as an eternal Ideal in the mind of God, and then (incarnated) in a finite subject" (57).

Turning to the portrayals of Christ in "the Epistles," Ward concludes that "Jesus manifests the ideal form of a perfected human life, fulfilled by conscious unity with the Spirit of God" (70). While this is true, Ward recognizes that Jesus is also "more than this," for he has "a destiny and reality much greater than his human form considered alone allows" on account of being "the heir, the ruler and disposer, of thousands of millions of galaxies" as the one who "will finally be sovereign over the whole cosmos" (70). Jesus Christ is not some personal Logos that has united itself to "an impersonal human nature" (74). Instead, he is a fully human person who perfectly actualizes the divine Ideal (that is "the Word").

Ward puts these pieces together when he discusses the "idea of the incarnation." Jesus Christ is fully human, and in this sense he shares our condition. But he is also "in some sense identical" with God. Thus there is an "absolute ontological uniqueness" to Jesus (74). As Ward explains, Jesus is unique in virtue of "being fully united to God from the first moment of earthly existence and in living by the full and unimpeded power of the Spirit" (74). Such union is possible only by a "unique divine initiative," but it is possible nonetheless (74–75). Indeed, in the person of Jesus Christ such union is not only possible but also actual.

So in Christ's "grace-perfected life," there is "no alienating distance between God's nature and this human nature." Therefore "one could rightly say that the acts of this human person accord perfectly with what God wills and with what God is." This "likeness is not accidental." To the contrary, it is "essential" (76–77). Ward summarizes his proposal:

> On this view, Jesus is a truly human person, but he is not only a human person. He is also, by what I have called a synergistic union, the earthly manifestation of God. There is the deepest possible unity, original and indissoluble, between his humanity and the mind and will of God. In that sense, Jesus is God. But he is not God *simpliciter*. He is God insofar as God turns towards the world in compassion and takes form within the world – God as participant in the world.   (78)

What are we to make of the prayers of Jesus to his Father? Ward says that "it is the human person of Jesus, who is truly in some sense identical with God as participant, who prays to God as creator" (78–79). And what does it mean to say that Jesus Christ is "in some sense identical?" Ward answers with an appeal to "double aspect identity theory" in philosophy of mind, and he concludes that "we could say that the human Jesus is identical to God in the following way: 'whatever it is' that unites both human and divine natures in Jesus forms one unitary reality, but within that unity two separate aspects can be distinguished—the finite and human, and the infinite and divine" (79). In Jesus "there is a compound unity of a human subject who expresses the eternal thought of God," and "the Word of God is the eternal ideal in the mind of God which Jesus will actualize on earth" (81).

So Ward recognizes that Jesus Christ is "in some sense both human and divine," and he works to give an account of what it means to affirm the humanity of Jesus. But what about the "divinity" of Christ? Does the grace-perfected union of this man with God "make Jesus divine" (81)? Well, as we have seen, it clearly does so "in some sense." But it just as clearly "does not confer omnipotence and omniscience" on Jesus (81). What we are left with is this: the incarnation "makes Jesus not only the realization of the divine ideal, but also the one through whom God acts decisively to liberate the world from the bondage of evil," thus Jesus is "both the revelation of the goal of union with God and the one who establishes the definitive Way to such union" (81). Therefore "Jesus is both uniquely God-with-us and the Saviour of the world" (81).

As Ward knows, there is considerable distance between his proposal and traditional doctrines of the Trinity and Incarnation (and even more distance from other recent revisionists such as Jürgen Moltmann). This is, after all, a "reformulation." Indeed, in some ways it is a radical reformulation, and we need to appreciate just how radical it is.

Traditional Christian doctrine holds that there is love shared between the Father and the Son within the Triune life.[42] Ward denies that there is such love within the "immanent Trinity" (e.g., x, 117–118, 186). Traditional doctrine maintains that one of the divine "persons," the pre-existent Logos who is the eternal Son of the Father, became fully and completely human without ceasing to be fully and completely divine. Ward denies that there was such a divine person to become incarnate. He denies that any pre-existent divine person became a "human primate" (xi). The broad Christian tradition has insisted that one of the three divine persons became human. "Concretists" have held that the Son took upon himself a concrete but not yet "hypostatized" individual human nature (and then have disagreed among themselves about the details), while "abstractists" have suggested that the Son took upon himself the set of properties individually necessary and jointly sufficient for being truly human. Despite their disagreements about the details of their proposals, however, both concretists and abstractists have held in common the deep conviction that the doctrine of the incarnation means that a distinct divine person who pre-existed his humanity took upon himself something that he did not have before—human nature.[43] Unless

---

[42] Even Thomas Aquinas, often taken to be the representative of "Latin" Trinitarian theology, insists that there is mutual love between the divine persons. See, e.g., *ST* 1a.37.2. See also the discussion in Gilles Emery, *The Trinitarian Theology of Thomas Aquinas* (Oxford: Oxford University Press, 2007), p. 155.

[43] For a brief overview of various concretist and abstractist strategies, see Thomas H. McCall, *An Invitation to Analytic Christian Theology* (Downers Grove: InterVarsity Academic, 2015), pp. 91–121.

I have badly misunderstood him, Ward denies all this. So we can conclude that this indeed is a rather radical "reformulation" of doctrine.

5.3.2 Theological Exegesis and Philosophical Theology

Happily, Ward engages in theological exegesis of the New Testament. As an exercise in analytic philosophical theology, his work is not devoid of attention to the biblical accounts that first gave rise to the formalized doctrine of the Trinity. He notes that "some theologians find evidence of three distinct individuals, who are all divine (three subjects of consciousness and will—Father, Son, and Spirit) in the Gospels" (33). Interestingly, he admits that "this is by no means an absurd suggestion" (33). But he ultimately rejects it in favor of an alternative interpretation of the Gospel accounts.

Before moving further, it is important to note that Ward repeatedly refers to the "social" doctrine that he rejects as positing three "individuals" (e.g., 33) who are "independent" (e.g., 63) or "self-existent" and "self-subsistent" (e.g., 53). But such descriptions do not adequately capture what most self-avowed proponents of ST are saying, and it overlooks or obscures the fact that many proponents of ST are actively trying to *overcome* what they take to be hyper-modern notions of individuality and autonomy. Indeed, as we have seen, many advocates of ST look to the doctrine of the Trinity precisely as a way to do so! So this is, at best, a misleading and pejorative way of putting matters. Many would agree with Ward's denial that the biblical basis for the doctrine of the Trinity supports such conclusions—but then go right ahead and promote ST as scripturally warranted. In other words, they might concur wholeheartedly—even enthusiastically—with Ward when he says that "there are reasons to doubt a 'three individuals' view of the Trinity" but maintain that this does nothing to settle the debates over ST (41). But having noted this, let us return to Ward's handling of the biblical passages. In keeping with my concern for the importance of Johannine theology for consideration of these issues, our primary attention will be there. But a few brief comments on Ward's engagement with other important New Testament themes and texts may be helpful.

When considering the Synoptic Gospels, Ward allows that these texts "give good reason for beginning to think of God as Trinity," but he denies that there is "a doctrine of a social Trinity in the Synoptic Gospels" (48). Of course it would be a stretch to argue that there is any full-blown or conceptually developed *doctrine* of the Trinity at all in the Synoptics, but is it the case that these accounts do not lend any support to a social account? As we have seen, Ward will allow that the Jesus of the New Testament is divine "in some sense," and he also recognizes that Jesus is distinct from his Father. But just *how* is Jesus distinct from his Father and, while clearly being fully and completely human, also different from other humans (e.g., 48)? Ward makes it obvious that he does *not* think that these texts teach that Jesus was pre-existent *as a person*—as an idea or ideal, yes, but not as a person who pre-exists his incarnation as human. It is understandable that Ward would not see elements supportive of a "social" view of the Trinity in the Synoptics, for biblical scholars have for decades held a similar view. However, he overstates the case, and he pays no attention whatsoever to the "I have come" statements of Jesus. When we take these seriously, however, we see that the gospel accounts portray Christ as the person who is the Son who has acted to become incarnate. As Simon Gathercole says, the Son "*acts* to take on human existence: though in the form of God, he *empties* himself to become incarnate."[44] We see similar themes when we look at Ward's consideration of "the Epistles." He briefly surveys some of the New Testament discussions of the Son and Spirit, and he concludes that "the New Testament, taken as a whole, thus speaks of God as a dynamic, creative, and relational reality, a reality known in a basic threefold relation to a created world" (72). Note carefully his statement that this is "to a created world"; it is "in the unfolding of history that God is Trinity" (72). Rather than an eternal and necessary Trinity, instead we have a God who becomes Triune in and through the acts of history. But Ward fails to interact with most of the key New Testament texts that have historically been used to establish both the divinity and distinction of the Son (and Spirit). There is no sustained treatment of, say, the deployment of the Shema in 1 Cor 8, or the citation of (Deutero-)Isaiah in Phil 2:5-11. And he offers no interaction with the serious New Testament scholarship that argues for the divinity of Christ in distinction from, and in relation to, his Father.[45]

Turning now to Ward's handling of the Johannine witness, Ward observes that the term "Logos" or "Word" is a "strangely impersonal term" that "does not seem to refer to a self-subsistent being, or one who exists as a person, in

---

[44] Simon Gathercole, *The Preexistent Son: Recovering the Christologies of Matthew, Mark, and Luke* (Grand Rapids: William B. Eerdmans Publishing Co., 2006), p. 290 (emphasis original).

[45] See Andrew Loke, *The Origin of Divine Christology* (Cambridge: Cambridge University Press, 2017); Chris Tilling, *Paul's Divine Christology* (Grand Rapids: William B. Eerdmans Publishing Co., 2015).

the sense of having a distinct and unique consciousness and agency" (53, cf. 55), and he concludes from the use of *theos* without a definite article (in John 1:1) that this likely means simply that "the Word was divine" but leaves the "exact form of identity with God indeterminate" (52–53). Because "Word" is an impersonal term, Ward denies that this is a "person" who pre-exists his incarnate humanity. Instead, it refers to a thought or an ideal (or, following C. H. Dodd, the "Platonic Idea of Man") (56). Jesus is thus "the Ideal made physical or given finite particularity" (56). Ward makes a valid point about the term itself, but his observation about the term itself is largely irrelevant to the issue at hand. For it is the *use* of the term that matters (rather than the "normal" or non-biblical uses of the term). And, as Bauckham points out, the context and usage of the term in John 1 makes a direct connection to the Genesis creation account: "the opening words 'In the beginning' (*en arche*) are identical with the opening of Genesis (Hebrew *beresit*, Greek LXX *en arche*)."[46] With this important background, we can see that "In the Prologue the evangelist uses 'Word' to identify the preexistent Christ *within the Genesis narrative*, and so within the unique identity of God *as already understood by Jewish monotheism*."[47] This means that the Logos is not merely "divine" in some vague and potentially lesser sense, for—according to the monotheism being affirmed—there is exactly one God. Following this unmistakable identification of the Logos, Johannine theology then refers to him as "Son"—which is unmistakable as an unambiguously personal term.[48]

Moreover, Ward's impersonal (or pre-personal) account of the pre-existence of the "Son" hardly does justice to the ample Johannine witness to Jesus's own statements of pre-existence. As Gathercole says, there is "an overwhelming *scholarly* consensus" that proper interpretation of Johannine theology leads us to conclude a clear doctrine of pre-existence.[49] As Ward himself admits, not only is it true that "the Father 'speaks' through Jesus, and Jesus 'sees' the Father," it is also true that "Jesus remembers that he pre-existed with God, was sent by God, and came down from heaven, 'where he was before' (John 6:62)" (54). After all, the incarnate Word is "the one who descended from heaven, the Son of Man" (John 3:13) (54). Thus, as Ward

---

[46] Richard Bauckham, "Monotheism and Christology in the Gospel of John," in Richard N. Longenecker ed., *Contours of Christology in the New Testament* (Grand Rapids: William B. Eerdmans Publishing Co., 2005), p. 150.

[47] Bauckham, "Monotheism and Christology," p. 151.

[48] See Bauckham, "Monotheism and Christology," p. 151.

[49] Simon Gathercole, *The Preexistent Son: Recovering the Christologies of Matthew, Mark, and Luke* (Grand Rapids: William B. Eerdmans Publishing Co., 2005), p. 83.

recognizes, "the Johannine Jesus knows that, as unfleshed Word which has now taken flesh in him, he existed with God in glory. It follows that when Jesus says 'I' in these Johannine speeches, he does not refer only to a human subject of action and experience" (55). But, on any acceptable criteria of identity, this "I" cannot be a mere ideal. If the Logos or Son speaks as a person about his pre-existent life with the Father, then the Logos or Son cannot have been less than personal in this pre-existent state. If Ward is right that "Jesus remembers" that "*he* pre-existed," then the "I" of the Johannine Jesus cannot merely be "this human subject, which is the image or perfect expression of the eternal thought of God" (57). If it is the *person* who is the *I*, and if this person can refer to himself as "I" in a pre-existent state, then this cannot be reducible to an instantiation of humanity that happens to conform perfectly to the divine Ideal. If the Word *is* the Son who *is* this Jesus of Nazareth, then this Word cannot merely be "an eternal possibility made actual, first as an eternal Ideal in the mind of God, and then (incarnate) in a finite subject" (57).

There is a curious lacuna in Ward's treatment of the Johannine materials. Jesus's "high priestly" prayer in John 17 is scarcely noticed, and it receives no sustained attention at all. As we have seen, he resolutely denies that there is love within the life of the (immanent) Trinity. Given God's creative action, we can speak rightly of divine love, and Ward can say that "the Trinity expresses the nature of God as love" (62). What he means is this: "the threefold form of love—as creating finite persons, relating in love to them, and uniting them to the divine life—is the manifestation (the 'exegesis,' John says in his prologue) of the supreme goodness of God as creative, self-giving, and universally inclusive love" (62). Ward refers to "the nature of God as love," but it is not clear what he means by this. Nor is it obvious that he can say this with consistency. If love is genuine, then presumably it is love for another and extends to the other. If he were to embrace a doctrine of God according to which love is essential to God's own intra-Trinitarian life, then he could do this with no problem. Without such a theology, however, love can only be essential to God if a created order of finite objects exists in relation to God. But Ward is very reticent to endorse such a speculative supposition, so it is not clear that he can with consistency hold that love is essential to God or part of the divine nature.[50]

---

[50] Thomas Jay Oord presses this point in "Can God Be Essentially Loving without Being Essentially Social? An Affirmation of and Alternative for Keith Ward," *Philosophia Christi* 18:2 (2016), pp. 353–361.

What is perhaps most striking in Ward's treatment of Johannine theology is his account of John 17. He refers to this prayer only as a statement about the "uniting of humans to the being of God" and the "unity of Father, Son, and believers" (63). He takes no notice of the fact that the unity of humans and God is based upon the prior and more fundamental unity of the Father and the Son.[51] And Ward somehow fails to even observe that this prayer of the incarnate Son is directed toward the Father who not only sent him into the world but who loved him "before the creation of the world" (John 17:24). The love is mutual, the love is expressed in personal indexicals (I-Thou), and the love is from before the foundation of the world. As mutual, it cannot be merely the words of Jesus's humanity. As personal, it cannot be merely instantiation of a divine ideal but instead is the love of a person for a person. And as eternal, it cannot be merely the temporally located statement of the fulfillment of the eternal possibility. In light of Johannine theology, it is safe to conclude that Ward's denial of intra-Trinitarian love is unwarranted. Indeed, we can say that if the evangelist of John's Gospel is right, then Ward is just simply wrong.

As I have pointed out, discussions of ST often suffer from a lack of clarity about just what it is that is being discussed. Despite its admirable clarity elsewhere, Ward's analytic treatment of the doctrine shares this defect. If by "ST" we mean something like (R-ST), then Ward may be more justified in his insistence that proper theological exegesis of the New Testament does not demand ST. But if he means something more like (L-ST) or (D-ST), then I think that we have grounds to conclude—with Ward—that a "'social' account of the Trinitarian God has a basis in the biblical writings" (42).

5.3.3 An Analysis of Ward's Christology

Ward knows, of course, that his theology is far removed from traditional doctrine in some important ways. He obviously doesn't think that this is a problem, and many sympathizers might think that the distance from traditional doctrine is a positive feature of his proposal. But several issues are puzzling, and some seem downright troublesome for his account.

Much of what Ward says about the incarnation could be taken as a fairly straightforward affirmation of a version of adoptionism or some other kind

---

[51] On which, see Grant MaCaskill, *Union with Christ in the New Testament* (Oxford: Oxford University Press, 2013), pp. 265–266.

of "Christology from below" (73–74). To say merely that Jesus Christ is man who actualizes God's ideal for humanity by his cooperation with God is fully consistent with adoptionism. And to add that Jesus becomes the "medium" through whom God achieves divine purposes ("through the absolute moral purity and inspired wisdom of Jesus") does not take us any further (74). If this were all that Ward has to say, then his proposal would be consistent with a Unitarian doctrine of God and an adoptionist Christology. If this were all that Ward had to say, then it might be more accurate to call his proposal "a reformulation of Unitarian doctrine." But this is not all that Ward has to say. For he also says that while Christ is a human person, he "is not only a human person" (78). Ward speaks of the "absolute ontological uniqueness" of Jesus (74), and (as we have seen), he insists further that Jesus Christ is divine "in some sense" (48)—and indeed that Christ is "in some sense identical with God" (78–79, 99).

5.3.3.1 Some Concerns about the "Identity" Claim

As we have seen, Ward holds that Jesus Christ is divine "in some sense," and indeed is "identical" with God "in some sense." Jesus, Ward says, "is presented in the Gospels as a man who is uniquely close to—so close as to be in some sense identical with—God" (73). But it is hard to know what to make of these claims. Proximity does not amount to identity, and it is simply a category mistake to claim that it is. Consider Ward's claim about the identity of Jesus: Jesus is divine "in some sense." What does this mean? Identity does not come in degrees. Now Ward is clear that the laws of logic really do apply to God. As he puts it, "Not only is the divine being conditioned by God's own necessary existence, knowledge, power, and goodness, but it is also conditioned by the existence of necessary truths in logic and morality" (164). So—thankfully—he will not simply hand-wave away any concerns about identity. And there *are* some concerns, for if we know anything about identity, we know that it does not come in degrees.

For if we know anything about identity, we know that identity is reflexive, transitive, and symmetric. We know that it is an equivalence relation that satisfies the well-known principle of the "Indiscernibility of Identicals":

(InId): $(\forall x)\ (\forall y)\ [x = y \Rightarrow (\forall P)\ (P(x) \Leftrightarrow P(y))]$

For any objects x and y, if x and y are identical, then for any property P, x has P if and only if y has P.

Accordingly, if the man Jesus Christ is identical with God, then for any property P had by the man Jesus Christ, that P is also had by God. And, of course, for any property P had by God, that P will also be had by the man Jesus Christ. So, if the man Jesus Christ is identical to God, and if the man Jesus Christ has the property of *beginning to exist in the first century*, then God began to exist in the first century. If the man Jesus Christ is identical with God, and if the man Jesus Christ has the property *died on a Roman cross in Jerusalem in the first century*, then God also died on a Roman cross in Jerusalem in the first century. We could multiply these examples readily, and in each case the conclusions would seem difficult for Ward to accept. For not only would identity entail the conclusion that God "looks like a human primate" (xi), we would be left with the conclusion that God indeed *is* (or, perhaps, *was*) a human primate. This seems to be exactly what Ward is trying to avoid.

In addition, if God is identical to the man Jesus Christ, and if God has the property *is the Creator of all humans*, then the man Jesus Christ also has the property *is the Creator of all humans*. But then the man Jesus Christ would be the Creator of all humans—and thus the Creator of himself. It is hard to see how this could be a welcome implication for Ward's view. Further, if God is identical to the man Jesus Christ, and if God has the properties of *being omniscient*, *being omnipotent*, and *being everlasting*, then the man Jesus Christ also has these properties. But Ward is insistent that the man Jesus Christ is *not* omnipotent or omniscient (81). So this implication cannot be welcome. Welcome or not, however, it is unavoidable. For according to (InId), it cannot be otherwise. Accordingly, the coherence of his project seems to be in jeopardy.

Of course it is no secret that such issues also raise worries for traditional Trinitarian theology and Christology.[52] The "logical problem of the Trinity" is well known, and what we know about identity raises concerns there too.[53] For if the Son *is* God (where the *is* is understood as identity), and if the Father *is* God (where the *is* is understood as identity), then—given transitivity—isn't the Father identical to the Son? That conclusion cannot be true according to orthodox Trinitarianism, but that conclusion also seems unavoidable for the proponents of orthodox Trinitarianism. Or so say the

[52] It is also no secret that traditional theology has resources to deal with such worries. But Ward rejects these traditional views, so he cuts himself off from their resources.

[53] See McCall and Rea, "Introduction," pp. 1–2.

critics. Awareness of such worries of incoherence have pushed theologians defending traditional formulations to formulate various theories. For instance, "Social Trinitarians" have taken the *is* to be the *is* of predication rather than the *is* of identity (and then have worked to avoid tritheism). The extent to which the various "Social Trinitarian" strategies are successful may be open to debate, but for present purposes we need not try to sort all that out here. We need not do so because Ward has vehemently rejected such proposals. Indeed, his rejection of them has been so thorough-going that he even rejects the "Latin Trinitarian" proposal of Brian Leftow for being too close to the "Social" views—this despite the fact that one would be hard pressed to find an analytic (Trinitarian) theologian who is a more forceful critic of ST than Leftow! So, in light of the fact that he has rejected it, we may safely conclude that ST does not present a way forward for Ward's proposal.

Some theologians who are dissatisfied with the various defensive strategies of ST appeal to the theory of "relative identity." Proponents of relative identity tend to think that (InId) is ill-formed; they hold that objects may be identical under one sortal concept but distinct under another sortal concept. As Michael C. Rea summarizes it, the theory of relative identity affirms both

(R1) statements of the form 'x = y' are incomplete and therefore ill-formed. A proper identity statement has the form 'x is the same F as y'

and

(R2) states of affairs of the following sort are possible: x is an F, y is an F, x is a G, y is a G, x is the same F as y, but y is not the same G as y.[54]

Applied to the doctrine of the Trinity, this strategy promises to safeguard a doctrine according to which there is exactly one God (in the numerical rather than merely generic sense of one), and according to which there are exactly three divine persons. For, as Peter van Inwagen says, "without classical identity, there is no absolute counting: there is only counting by Ns."[55] Accordingly, when we are counting "divine Beings by beings, there is one; counting divine Persons by beings, there is one; counting divine Beings by persons, there are three; counting divine Persons by persons, there are

[54] Michael C. Rea, "Relative Identity and the Doctrine of the Trinity," *Philosophia Christi* 5 (2003), p. 434.
[55] Peter van Inwagen, *God, Knowledge, and Mystery: Essays in Philosophical Theology* (Ithaca: Cornell University Press, 1995), p. 250.

three."[56] Could Ward appeal to "Relative Trinitarianism" as a resource, and would it help his view regain coherence?

It is less than obvious that this strategy holds much hope for his proposal. Rea raises a worry: anyone who is committed to the truth of the doctrine of relative identity and who also holds that the words "is God" and "is distinct from" should be understood in this way might encounter problems that are nothing short of "catastrophic" and "disastrous."[57] For such a strategy opens the door to anti-realism, the critics worry, and at best it gives quarter to modalism. Given Ward's desire to avoid modalism, this does not look like a promising way out.

Rea also argues that an "impure" version (which does not endorse some doctrine of relative identity but only claims that the words "is God" and "is distinct from" express relativized identity and distinctness relations rather than absolute identity and distinctness relations) can work if one tells a "supplementary story to explain the metaphysics" of these relations.[58] He then (with Jeffrey E. Brower) appropriates an account of material constitution to tell that supplementary story. On this account, the "is" (of the statement that "the Son is God" and "the Father is God") is the "is" of numerical (and indeed essential rather than accidental) sameness (rather than merely being the "is" of predication), but it is not the "is" of identity. Appealing to the analogy of hylomorphic compounds and applying this to the doctrine of the Trinity, Brower and Rea conclude that there are three divine persons who are really distinct and fully divine while there is exactly one God.[59]

Might Ward appeal to such a solution? He says things that might indicate that he is sympathetic to such a strategy. For instance, he objects to David Wiggins's claims about absolute identity, and when he refers to the Athanasian Creed he insists that "the 'is' here is not the 'is' of strict identity." Instead, he says, "It is an 'is' of inclusion" (239) (unfortunately, he does not interact at all with the strategies of either van Inwagen, on the one hand, or Brower-Rea or William Hasker on the other hand). So he seems sympathetic, and, at any rate, this seems like the most hopeful way forward for this proposal. But it is not clear that he can help himself to this strategy—at

---

[56] van Inwagen, *God, Knowledge, and Mystery*, p. 250.
[57] Rea, "Relative Identity and the Doctrine of the Trinity," pp. 442–443.
[58] Rea, "Relative Identity and the Doctrine of the Trinity," p. 442.
[59] Jeffrey E. Brower and Michael C. Rea, "Material Constitution and the Trinity," *Faith and Philosophy* 22:1 (2005), p. 69.

least not with any consistency.[60] For on the Brower-Rea proposal, the divine persons share numerical sameness that is "*essential* sameness." But on Ward's theology, this is less than secure, since Jesus Christ is essentially divine only "in some sense." This brings us to concerns about the divinity of Christ.

5.3.3.2 Some Questions about the Divinity of Christ

Recall that Ward insists that Christ really is "divine"—though only "in some sense" (e.g., 81). Just what sense is that? What does it mean to say that some being is "divine in some sense?" The answers to these questions are less than pellucid, but what is obvious is Ward's frank denial that Jesus Christ is omnipotent and omniscient (81). He is the "realization of the divine ideal" (81) that is eternally possible but actualized in this man, and Jesus is the "one through whom God acts decisively to liberate the world from the bondage of evil" (81). He is divine; he is God-with-us. But he isn't omnipotent.

So however exactly we are to take it, we do know that Ward denies that the Jesus who is "uniquely God-with-us" (81) is omnipotent and omniscient. Jesus is divine "in some sense," thus he must have the divine essence "in some sense." But he isn't omniscient or omnipotent. So just how are we to understand this? When we take into account what Ward says about the identity of Jesus (and the identity of God), it is not plausible to take the claim of "essence" in the sense of individual-essence. So, apparently, we should take the essence claim to be a claim about a kind-essence. Taking the essence to be a kind-essence, then the divine essence is something like the "full set of properties, individually necessary and jointly sufficient" for being God.

Accordingly, I take it that the most plausible way to interpret Ward is this: the divine essence is the set of properties or attributes that are "necessary" for God (knowledge, power, and goodness, etc.) (164). Notably, omnipotence is to be ascribed to God; it is part of the divine essence (165). But when we consider Jesus, we are told that he is *not* omnipotent (81). What are we to make of this? So far as I can see, it leaves us with nothing short of the conclusion that there are different divine essences. There is God's divine

---

[60] Moreover, if he were to allow that such a strategy works to defend the traditional formulations, then he would unable to reject what he calls "Social Trinitarianism" with such hand-waving. For if some "relative identity" strategy works, then it seems that it can also work (as it does for van Inwagen) to maintain belief in both *one God* and *three persons* (where "person" is understood in a robust sense). So accepting some version of relative identity might be bad news overall for Ward's project, as it would undercut the major motivation for his revisionist theology.

essence, and this includes the attribute of omnipotence. There is also, apparently, the divine essence of the Son, and this does not include omnipotence. So God has an omnipotence-rich divine essence (call it the O-positive divine essence), while Jesus Christ has an omnipotence-less divine essence (call it the O-negative divine essence).

But if one has the O-positive divine essence and the other has an O-negative divine essence, then it is obvious that they have different essences. How would this not entail that there are different *gods*? If Jesus is "divine" but not omnipotent, then he is of a different divinity. Indeed, he is of a weaker or lesser divinity. If he is of a different divinity, then it is obvious that he is a different God. And if he is of a lesser divinity, then he it is just as clear that he is not only a different "God" but also a *lesser* "God." In his opposition to "Social Trinitarianism," Ward is convinced that three divine persons (who are distinct centers of consciousness and will) would be three gods. As Ward sees things, saying that they are all of the same divine essence (understood as a generic or kind-essence) is no help (or at least not enough help), for this only yields three Gods of the same kind. But how is it any better to have two Gods *of different kinds*? Isn't that still, by Ward's accounting or anyone else's, two Gods? And, for Ward or any other non-polytheist, isn't that exactly one God too many? The defender of Ward may remonstrate that there is only one of the "high" God; that is, there is only one God with O-positive divinity. But even if we are supposing that this is true, that doesn't tell us that there is only one God. It merely says that there is one of *that* kind of God, one O-positive God. Again, if we have one O-positive God and one O-negative God, we nonetheless have two Gods. For anyone who wants to avoid polytheism, surely that is one God too many.

Shorn of the claims that Christ is divine "in some sense" and identical with God "in some sense," Ward's proposal would be rigorously monotheistic—but it would also be at odds with what he recognizes to be the New Testament witness to Christ. Fascinating and innovative though it is, his proposal really wouldn't be a reformulation of *Trinitarian* doctrine as much as it would be a recommendation of *Unitarian* theology. *With* those claims about Christ's divinity and identity, however, the coherence of Ward's fascinating proposal is called into question. Indeed, without further clarification (or correction), we are left to wonder why Ward's proposal wouldn't turn out to be a very erudite and sophisticated recommendation of a rather unusual form of polytheism.

5.3.4 Conclusion

In this section I have introduced Ward's creative proposal of a robustly anti-Social Trinitarian doctrine of God. After surveying the approach and summarizing his conclusions, I then engaged with his theological exegesis. This in turn led to a theological analysis of his own constructive proposal. We have seen that his opposition to ST is so deep and so pronounced that he both denies love within the intra-Trinitarian life of God and even the real personal pre-existence of the Son. He is convinced that love within the Trinity would entail or equate a version of ST, and he is concerned that to allow for truly personal pre-existence is to give up the game. Thus he rejects both.

I have argued that his theological exegesis both commits several mistakes in dealing with the texts with which it engages and ignores other passages which are of critical importance. As a result, his doctrine is under-supported by Scripture and indeed must be judged at odds with some important texts. Beyond this, his own constructive doctrine is beset with problems. If he were to reject any affirmation of the divinity of Christ, then his position would be consistent. It would be a version of Unitarianism, but it would be consistent. But with his affirmations that Jesus Christ is divine "in some sense"—but without an adequate account of just what that sense *is*—it appears that his version may entail the very dogma that he most wants to avoid. For it is unclear that he is able to escape worries of polytheism.

5.4 The Communion of the Father and the Son: A Closer Look

So, as we have seen, Ward rejects ST. Because he is convinced that this would allow or entail tritheism, he rejects any recognition of the love of the (immanent) Trinity and indeed any affirmation of the personal pre-existence of the eternal Son. Ward may be the most thorough-going of ST's critics, but he is far from alone. But is he right—does the recognition of mutual love within the Trinity entail ST? And is ST so obviously guilty of tritheism?

5.4.1 The Love of the Father for the Son

Many theologians have been convinced that a close reading of Johannine theology leads us directly to the conclusion that the Father and Son share mutual love. As Marianne Meye Thompson says, the Fourth Gospel makes it clear that the Father "loves the Son (5:20; 10:17; 15:9; 17:23, 26)."[61] The love of the Father and Son for one another is deemed "programmatic" in John's account.[62] For instance, in his famous "high priestly prayer," Jesus offers us a precious glimpse into the intra-Triune life (sans incarnation). Here he prays to his Father, and here he refers to the love of the Father for the Son "before the creation of the world" (John 17:24). As Thompson observes, the "Father has loved the Son 'before the world came to be' (17:5), before the 'foundation of the world' (v. 24)"; this love "has always characterized the relationship of Father and Son."[63] "Indeed," she says, "the mutual love of the Father and the Son lies at the heart of their relationship (3:35; 5:20; 10:17)."[64] Perhaps even more astounding than the insight that there is love *within* the Father-Son relationship apart from the creation of the world is what follows: Jesus prays that those who know him are loved by the Father *even as* the Father loves the Son (John 17:23), and he prays that the love that the Father has for the Son "may be in them" (John 17:26). Johannine theology goes on to make several similar affirmations: not only does God love the world (e.g., John 3:16), but God *is* love (1 John 4:8). Thompson argues that the "unity of Father and Son is described, not only as mutual indwelling ("you in me and I in you," 17:21), but also in terms of love for each other."[65] This love, which is "self-giving, not self-seeking, is cohesive."[66] She concludes that this intra-divine love "is not one of the many possible attributes or actions that the Father may express towards the Son, the Son towards the Father and believers, and so on," rather "it is the fundamental way of relating among those who find their very life and existence determined by the relationship of 'father' and 'son' to each other."[67] The Father loves the Son and the Son loves the Father—and this same love is now extended toward others. As D. A. Carson says, this "thought is breathtakingly extravagant."[68]

---

[61] Marianne Meye Thompson, *The God of the Gospel of John* (Grand Rapids: William B. Eerdmans Publishing Co., 2001), p. 69. She notes that this affirmation marks a distinction between the Fourth Gospel and the Synoptic depictions, pp. 98–99.

[62] Thompson, *The God of the Gospel of John*, p. 99.

[63] Marianne Meye Thompson, *John: A Commentary* (Louisville: Westminster John Knox Press, 2015), p. 357.

[64] Thompson, *The God of the Gospel of John*, p. 70.   [65] Thompson, *John*, p. 356.

[66] Thompson, *John*, p. 356.   [67] Thompson, *The God of the Gospel of John*, p. 100.

[68] D. A. Carson, *The Gospel According to John* (Grand Rapids: William B. Eerdmans Publishing Co., 1991), p. 569.

Andreas J. Kostenberger and Scott R. Swain insist that "John's account of Jesus's identity and mission is literally trinitarian from beginning to end."[69] This is anything but an idiosyncratic interpretation of the Johannine texts, and it is far from uniquely "modern" as a theological position. For instance, consider the legacies of two major medieval theologians whose views have enjoyed great influence: Richard of St. Victor and Thomas Aquinas. They clearly employ differing accounts of divine personhood. Richard holds that a divine person is an "incommunicable existence of a divine nature" (*persona divina est divinae naturae incommunicabilis existentia*).[70] Thomas, on the other hand, opts for what is basically a Boethian notion of person as "individual substance of a rational nature" (*persona est individua substantia rationalis naturae*).[71] Their views are distinct, and their legacies are disparate, with Henry of Ghent and John Duns Scotus notably following Richard's theology (and, at least in the case of Scotus, adjusting the doctrine of divine simplicity too).[72] Nonetheless, both affirm that love is of the essence of God—and both are convinced that the divine persons love one another in mutual fellowship and communion. As Richard puts it, within the simplicity of the divine life, being is identical to loving.[73] Thus Richard famously argues that perfect love is shared between the persons of the Trinity—and indeed mounts a kind of Anselmian argument for belief in the Trinity. The mutual love of the persons of the Trinity for one another is the *greatest* mutual love (the *summa condilectione*).[74] He concludes that this love is that greater than which and better than which cannot be conceived.[75] And Thomas does not differ from him on this point at all: "The Father and the Son love each other

[69] Andreas J. Kostenberger and Scott R. Swain, *Father, Son, and Holy Spirit: The Trinity and John's Gospel* (Downers Grove: InterVarsity Academic, 2008), p. 165.

[70] Richard of St. Victor, *De Trinitate* IV.xxii; *PL* 196 945C. This is in deliberate contradistinction to the definition of Boethius, e.g., *De Trinitate* IV.xxi; *PL* 196 945A.

[71] E.g., Thomas Aquinas, *Summa Theologica* Ia QQ29.1.

[72] E.g., *Henry of Ghent's Summa, Articles 53–55, On the Divine Persons*, translated and edited by Roland J. Teske, SJ (Milwaukee: Marquette University Press, 2015), pp. 94–96. See the helpful discussion in Richard A. Muller, *Post-Reformation Reformed Dogmatics: The Rise and Development of Reformed Orthodoxy, ca. 1520 to ca. 1725, Volume Four: The Triunity of God* (Grand Rapids: Baker Academic, 2003), pp. 50–54.

[73] Richard of St. Victor, *De Trinitate* V.xx; *PL* 196 963C-D; see also *Trinity and Creation*, Victorine Texts in Translation: Exegesis, Theology, and Spirituality from the Abbey of St. Victor, Boyd Taylor Coolman and Dale M. Coulter, eds. (New York: New City Press, 2011), pp. 312–313.

[74] Richard of St. Victor, *De Trinitate* III.xix; *PL* 196 927C; see also the translation in *Trinity and Creation: A Selection of Works of Hugh, Richard, and Adam of St. Victor*, pp. 262–263.

[75] Richard of St. Victor, *De Trinitate* III.ii; *PL*196 917A. Within God there is "*una voluntas, una charitas, una et indifferens bonitas*" as well as "*idem amor,*" *De Trinitate* V.xxiii, *PL* 196:963C. See *Trinity and Creation*, p. 315.

and love us by the Holy Spirit."[76] For there is a "twofold unity of the Father and the Son: a unity of essence and of love."[77] As Gilles Emery says, "We need not contrast Thomas's metaphysical attitude to the topic with one that stresses the 'psychological' elements of the person (such as the life of the mind: knowledge, freedom, action, and openness to another), because these elements are integrated into his own approach."[78] Dominic Legge says takes Aquinas's theology to mean that "this knowledge and love of Christ that the Holy Spirit gives is equally a knowledge and love of each of the divine persons, granting us a participation in the very inner life of the Trinity."[79]

Other major medieval theologians concur; as Marilyn McCord Adams describes the theology of John Duns Scotus, "God is a maximally-organized lover. The persons of the Trinity love one another with friendship love (*amor amicitiae*), which is unselfish and so reaches out to desire other co-lovers for the Beloved."[80]

More could be said, but such examples should show that the affirmation of intra-Trinitarian love is to be found across lines of disagreement—and, indeed, that this affirmation is to be seen even in the theology of the theologian often considered to be the "high-water mark" of Latin scholasticism. And this is found throughout the tradition for very good reason—many theologians have been convinced that this is where our Lord Jesus himself leads us.

So the Christian—at least the Christian who wishes to maintain contact with the broad tradition of creedal orthodoxy and who wishes to hold a view consistent with Johannine theology—should affirm that love is essential to the intra-Trinitarian life of God. Does this mean that she must affirm ST? And does this ST entail tritheism as Ward alleges? Well, if we take the proper definition (either in part or in whole) of ST to be (L-ST), then of course the affirmation that there is mutual love between Father and Son within the eternal Triune life just *is* ST. On the other hand, if we take a better

---

[76] E.g., Aquinas, *Summa Theologica* Ia.37.2. See also the helpful discussion of Gilles Emery, "The Trinity," in Eleonore Stump and Brian Davies, eds., *The Oxford Handbook of Aquinas* (Oxford: Oxford University Press, 2012), p. 423.

[77] Thomas Aquinas, *Commentary on the Gospel of John Chapters 9–21*, translated by Fr. Fabian R. Larcher, OP (Lander, WY: The Aquinas Institute for the Study of Sacred Doctrine, 2013), p. 380.

[78] Gilles Emery, *The Trinitarian Theology of St Thomas Aquinas* (Oxford: Oxford University Press, 2007), p. 106.

[79] Dominic Legge, OP, *The Trinitarian Christology of St Thomas Aquinas* (Oxford: Oxford University Press, 2017), p. 229.

[80] Marilyn McCord Adams, *What Sort of Human Nature? Medieval Philosophy and the Systematics of Christology* (Milwaukee: Marquette University Press, 1999), p. 69.

definition of ST and adopt (R-ST), then there is no good reason to think that this amounts to ST. Perhaps it is necessary for ST, but the affirmation of intra-Trinitarian love is not sufficient.

Either way, whether we adopt (L-ST) or hold out for (R-ST), there is no reason to think that the affirmation of intra-Trinitarian love qualifies as tritheism. For either way, there are multiple strategies available to those who wish to avoid the bogeyman of tritheism. There is more than one route open to the theologian who makes our affirmations: there are strategies for "modified ST," there are accounts of "numerical sameness without identity" (including those that appeal to the analogy of material constitution), and there is the possibility of retrieval of distinctly traditional "Latin" versions of the doctrine that can readily affirm this as well.[81]

5.4.2 The Father-Son Communion and the Issue of Agency

What is implied by an affirmation of intra-Trinitarian love? How should we think about the distinction of the persons? Are the Father and Son distinct *in agency*? Is the Father a distinct person from the Son in the sense of being an "I" in relation to another "Thou?" Are they, or do they have, distinct "centers of consciousness"?

As we have seen, the mainstream Christian tradition has been clear that divine action "outside of God" is always unified and undivided. As traditional Latin formulations put it, the *opera ad extra sunt omnia indivisa*. As long as this is properly understood, there is no reason that the theologian who recognizes the biblical witness to the reality of intra-Trinitarian love and who affirms it as such cannot affirm the traditional dictum as well. But what does it mean to understand it properly? Well, perhaps it will help to clear away a possible misunderstanding. The traditional dictum does not mean that there is no distinction in the divine action. To be "undivided" does not mean "indistinguishable." And not only is it true (for the mainstream Latin tradition) that the works of God *ad extra* are undivided, it is also true that these works of God can rightly be said to reach their *terminus* on one or another of the divine persons. It is basic to Christian orthodoxy—going all the way back to the rejection of patripassianism—that the Father does not become incarnate, does not suffer, and does not die. Nor does the

---

[81] E.g., Scott Williams, "Indexicals and the Trinity: Two Non-Social Models," *Journal of Analytic Theology* 1 (2013), pp. 74–94.

Spirit. Instead, "one of the Trinity suffered in the flesh." Only one of the divine persons, that is, actually became incarnate. So we should think of divine action as unified and undivided, but we should not think of it as undifferentiated. A better way of understanding the claim that the *opera ad extra* are undivided is offered by important theologians in the tradition. As Maximus the Confessor puts it, the Father and the Holy Spirit "themselves did not become incarnate, but the Father approved and the Spirit cooperated when the Son himself effected his incarnation."[82] John of Damascus takes a similar line: "the Father and the Holy Spirit take no part at all in the incarnation of the Word except in connection with the miracles, and in respect of good will and purpose."[83] So does Peter Lombard when he says that "it was specifically in the hypostasis of the Son, not jointly in the three persons, that divine nature united the human one to itself."[84]

When we consider the *opera ad intra*, however, matters are rather different. Here the work of the Father is entirely distinct from that of the Son. For on traditional doctrine, the Father generates the Son—and *only* the Father generates the Son. Whatever exactly eternal generation *is* may be rather mysterious, but, whatever exactly it is, it is something that only the Father does. The Son does not generate himself. Indeed, on some accounts of the internal relations, the "relations of opposition" are the only real distinctions between the person (*ad intra*). So there is a sense in which the works of one divine person are entirely distinct from those of the other divine persons. Thus it seems not unreasonable to conclude that their agency is distinct in some sense. Indeed, as Scott Williams concludes, the traditional view is that while "some acts are shared among the persons," it is also true that "some acts distinguish the divine persons. Only the Father begets the Son."[85]

The New Testament depiction of the relationships between the divine persons leaves little room for doubt about the distinction. The Father uses "I" in relation to the Son (Matt 3:17). The Son uses "I" in relation to the Father (e.g., John 17:1-24). So, if we practice theological interpretation of Scripture and understand the biblical narratives to be referring to the *Triune*

---

[82] Maximus the Confessor, *On the Lord's Prayer PG* 90:876. I employ the translation used in Richard Swinburne's *The Christian God* (Oxford: Oxford University Press, 1994), p. 181 n7.

[83] John of Damascus, *De Fide Orthodoxa* III.11 *NPNF* 9:55.

[84] Peter Lombard, *Sentences, Book Three: On the Incarnation of the Word*, trans. Guilio Silano (Toronto: Pontifical Institute of Medieval Studies, 2008), p. 21; *PL* 192:766.

[85] Scott Williams, "In Defense of a Latin Social Trinity: A Response to William Hasker," *Faith and Philosophy* 27 (2010), p. 10.

God, then we seem to have grounds to conclude that there is a robustly "I-Thou" relationship between Father and Son. Some critics may protest that this move comes too quickly. For if we interpret the New Testament theologically, and, following the tradition, understand it to be referring the Triune God, then we should also follow that same tradition and understand that these same personal indexicals refer to the *incarnate* Son. In other words, the critics might aver, these texts refer not to the Son *simpliciter* but to the Son incarnate *as the human Jesus Christ*. In other words, they might remonstrate, it is not simply "the Son" who is the referent of these dialogues but "the Son qua-humanity."

There is a long and venerable tradition to thinking this way about the incarnate Son: the God-human is to be understood not merely as human or divine but as human and divine. Since the human nature is not "confused" with the divine nature, we are to understand some things to be true of the Son qua or according to his human nature while understanding other things to be true of and appropriately predicated of the Son *qua* or according to his divine nature.

But whatever we think of this strategy in Christology—and it is beyond the scope of this chapter to pass judgment at this point—it does not change anything about the main point that I am making here. Even if we say that it is the Son qua-humanity who is the referent of the "I" in relation to the Father who is the "Thou," it is nonetheless true that it is *the Son* qua-humanity who is the referent. For it is not the humanity that is the referent. The humanity itself is *anhypostatic*. It is only the humanity joined to the person of the Son in the incarnation that is *enhypostatic* or "hypostatized." The humanity itself is not a distinct agent. The humanity itself is not a knower or doer. The humanity itself is not an "I" that somehow functions alongside of or in addition to the real person that is the eternal Son. Unless we are prepared to embrace a Nestorian Christology, the human nature cannot be considered as a personal entity in and of itself. So even if we say that these personal indexicals refer to the Son qua-humanity (or qua-human nature), it is still the case that it is *the Son*—rather than the Father or the Spirit—who is incarnate. Thus it is the Son—and not the Father or the Spirit—who is the referent of whatever is to be predicated of God qua-humanity.

As we have seen, Ward is sure that prayer is a merely human activity. He admits that "while the fact that Jesus prays to the Father distinguishes Jesus from the Father, it does not seem to reflect a distinction between two persons of the same sort."[86] For "it is Jesus as a dependent human being who prays to a being of much greater power," and "it is the suffering and limited human subject, included in the Word though it is, who prays to the Creator."[87] Similarly, Holmes insists that "prayer is necessarily a creaturely action."[88] But neither Ward nor Holmes gives us any sustained argument for this conclusion; instead it seems to serve as a presupposition that then functions as the premise of an argument. However, since this is the very issue at stake, to do so without further argument is to risk begging the question. On the other hand, it is not only Jesus who addresses his Father, for the Spirit also "intercedes" for creatures (Rom 8:26). Clearly, the Spirit is not incarnate. So the intercession of the Spirit cannot be counted as something to be taken qua-humanity. Unless the Spirit is a creature, then it seems that intercession is not merely a creaturely action.

In an important contribution to the contemporary discussions, Scott Williams works to retrieve some insights from the medieval Latin tradition. He offers what he refers to alternatively as "soft Latin Trinitarianism" or "Latin Social Trinitarianism." It is "Social" in the sense that the divine persons love one another, and it is social in the further sense that there are three divine agents. As Williams puts it, "there are three metaphysical agents (Father, Son, and Holy Spirit)."[89] And it is "Latin" in the sense that it follows the mainstream Latin tradition in recognizing both the real distinction of the divine persons and the numerical sameness of the divine being.[90] He observes that there is much more diversity in the scholastic Latin tradition than is sometimes recognized, and he makes a strong case for a distinctly "Franciscan" account that follows the lead of Richard of St. Victor. On this account, a "person" is an "incommunicable existent of an intellectual nature," and "each divine person is constituted by two items: the one and only one instance of the divine nature and an incommunicable personal attribute" (e.g., *begetting*).[91] Each divine person is irreducible to the other two, and the unique identity of each divine person is found only in relation to the others. At the same time, however, they share the numerically same instance of the divine nature (which is the *only* instance of the divine nature).

---

[86] Ward, *Christ and the Cosmos*, p. 40.   [87] Ward, *Christ and the Cosmos*, p. 40.

[88] Stephen R. Holmes, "Response to Thomas H. McCall," p. 142.

[89] Scott Williams, "Indexicals and the," p. 84. This is in marked and intentional contrast to Brian Leftow's "hard" Latin account according to which there is "one divine agent, God", p. 83.

[90] Williams, "Indexicals and the Trinity," p. 84.

[91] Williams, "Indexicals and the Trinity," p. 84.

Williams also argues, however, that the situation regarding the indexical "I" is rather more complicated than it might appear at first glance. Drawing on recent work by David Kaplan and John Perry, he draws a distinction between "utterances" and "tokens": utterances are intentional acts of communication, while tokens are "traces left by utterances" and can include speech, writing, symbols, or other gestures.[92] Following Perry, Williams argues that the numerically same token can be used to express different propositions. The various meanings are relative to the different contexts, thus one placard with the words "Vote for Bush" or "I support President Bush" may be used to communicate very different things. Notably, although there is one token, there are different meanings on both ends: the referent of "Bush" may change, and the referent of "I" may change. In Williams's summary

> we see that the referent of an indexical expression like "I," and the proposition entailed by it, depends upon the person *using* the token of "I." Moreover, an indexical expression like "I" *automatically* refers to the person using it. Lastly, we see that *numerically the same* token of an expression can be relative to diverse contexts and so can be used to affirm diverse propositions.[93]

The "referent and content of 'I'" are relative to the situation; they "are determined by the agent using the token," thus "The Son's using this token entails that the 'I' refers to the Son and not to the Father."[94] Accordingly, when the person who is the Father says "I am the Father," that person uses this token to say that he is identical with the Father. If, however, the person who is Son uses the same token, he uses it to mean that he is numerically the same God as the Father but not the person of the Father. The upshot is this: to have a robustly Trinitarian account of mutual love, one need not insist that "self-conscious acts" are "essential to person-hood even if the aptitude for such acts were implied," and if one wishes to retain only one "I" within the Trinity, then one can do so while maintaining belief in the genuine personal distinctions and even agency of the Father, Son, and Holy Spirit.[95]

[92] Williams, "Indexicals and the Trinity," p. 80.
[93] Williams, "Indexicals and the Trinity," pp. 82–83.
[94] Williams, "Indexicals and the Trinity," p. 85.
[95] Williams, "Indexicals and the Trinity," p. 90.

In an ongoing discussion with William Hasker, Williams is pressed to clarify various aspects of his proposal. Williams recognizes that his "Latin Social model" needs nuance on the matter of whether there is one divine consciousness rather than three of these. He distinguishes between three types of consciousness. What he calls "experiential consciousness" is the "what-it-is-like" consciousness. What he dubs "access consciousness" is "basic awareness of something such that one can interact with that thing." And what he refers to as "introspective consciousness" is "awareness of one's own awareness of something."[96] Armed with these distinctions, Williams maintains that the divine persons hold all their mental tokens in common while also allowing that one divine person's consciousness may differ from another in some respects. Thus their respective understandings of, say, "God the Father is wise" may not differ at all, but their introspective awareness of, say, "I am wise" will be differentiated. "So, God the Father knows what it is like to know that he (i.e., the Father) is wise; likewise, God the Son knows what it is like to know he (i.e., the Son) is wise, and God the Holy Spirit knows what it is like to know he (i.e., the Holy Spirit) is wise."[97] As Williams explains, in cases of contingent divine action—such as the divine Son becoming incarnate rather than the Father or Spirit—"what is shared is numerically the same act of using a divine mental token." But what "is not shared is exactly the same access consciousness (the proposition of which each is aware), experiential consciousness (what it's like to be aware of the proposition of which one is aware), and introspective consciousness (one's being aware of something about oneself)."[98]

In cases referring not to contingent divine action but to necessary truths related to the personal properties (such as the eternal generation of the Son), matters are even more clear-cut. So the Father "has experiential consciousness of what it's like to beget the Son and is introspectively conscious of his begetting the Son," and, since this pertains to the Father's incommunicable property, then this is a case of "experiential consciousness and introspective consciousness [that] cannot be shared with the Son (or Holy Spirit)."[99]

This analysis yields the following conclusion: "depending on the divine mental token being used and the proposition of which each person is aware, the persons are conscious of exactly the same thing or are conscious of

---

[96] Williams, "In Defense of a Latin Social Trinity," p. 11.
[97] Williams, "In Defense of a Latin Social Trinity," p. 12.
[98] Williams, "In Defense of a Latin Social Trinity," p. 12.
[99] Williams, "In Defense of a Latin Social Trinity," p. 13.

something different."[100] And all of this is consistent with there being exactly one divine substance, for on this account we have numerical sameness without identity. What we have then, are *multiple* ways to affirm the reality of mutual love within the Triune life as well as careful and sophisticated accounts of Trinitarian agency while also retaining belief in the numerical sameness of the Triune God. Thus we need not resort to (R-ST) to affirm the biblical witness to the union and communion of the Father, Son, and Holy Spirit. Whether or not such versions of ST are preferable in an all-things-considered sense is a topic for another day. But what should be clear at this point is that the common, generic-essence versions of Social Trinitarianism are not required to make the theological affirmations required by a proper understanding of the biblical witness.

5.5 Conclusion

As we have seen, Richard Bauckham is certain that Johannine theology supports ST. He contrasts ST with "much of the tradition," which is said to give "priority to the one divine substance over the three Persons in God" and instead holds that the "three Persons are irreducible."[101] I think that Bauckham is mistaken in claiming that (much of) the tradition prioritizes the substance over the persons in this way. This is not the place for an extended argument about such a claim, but my observations to this point about major figures in the Latin scholastic tradition (e.g., Richard of St. Victor) should at least provide some counter-evidence. But we should not be distracted by the historical claims and thus miss the constructive point. For surely Bauckham is correct to say that Johannine theology supports the central claim (made with emphasis by the defenders of ST) that the divine persons are irreducible—either to one another or to the divine substance. He is also right when he says that Johannine theology brings us to the conclusion that the "divine Persons are acting and relating subjects" and further that the concept of coinherence or perichoresis is "of critical importance."[102]

In this chapter I have engaged with the provocative proposal offered by Keith Ward as a way into broader considerations pertaining to the communion of love shared between Father and Son within the Holy Trinity. After working to sort out various conceptions (and misconceptions) of the label

[100] Williams, "In Defense of a Latin Social Trinity," p. 14.
[101] Bauckham, *Gospel of Glory*, p. 37.   [102] Bauckham, *Gospel of Glory*, p. 37.

"ST," I turned attention to the significant alternative to it offered by Ward. Here I introduced his position as well as his arguments against ST and for his own position. I argued that the case for his proposal is incomplete and flawed with respect to the theological exegesis of relevant biblical passages; here I noted some shortcomings with his own exegetical case and presented a counter-argument that appeals to Johannine theology. After offering some theological analysis of Ward's constructive proposal, I argued, contra Ward, that we both can and should affirm that there is mutual love within the Trinity. This much, at least, is a basic theological desiderata. We need not—although we can—resort to (R-ST) to affirm it. But Christian theologians who take the Johannine depiction to be a window—however shadowy and narrow it may be—into the life of the triune God should not hesitate to confess that God *is* love.

6

The Logos and His Logic

6.1 Introduction

"A contradiction is false. It is false everywhere and always. It is false in hell. It is false in heaven. It is even false in theology." With these words, a distinguished philosopher began a lecture to a group of divinity school students. Accustomed to quick and easy appeals to "mystery," the theology students and aspiring pastors before him were rather taken aback, but this statement reflects a view that is not uncommon among philosophers. Indeed, Graham Priest refers to classical logic and its commitment to the principles of non-contradiction and excluded middle as "orthodoxy."[1]

But in a recent and very important proposal for Christology, Jc Beall wields the resources of subclassical (or paraconsistent) logic in defense of Chalcedonian Christology.[2] The past few decades have seen much ink spilled and many trees killed in arguments over the coherence of orthodox Christology.[3] Critics such as John Hick have made the case that "to say,

---

[1] Graham Priest, Koji Tanaka, and Zach Weber, "Paraconsistent Logic," in Edward Zalta, ed., *Stanford Encyclopedia of Philosophy*, <https://plato.stanford.edu/archives/win2012/entries/davidson/>.

[2] Originally in Jc Beall, "Christ—A Contradiction: A Defense of Contradictory Christology," *Journal of Analytic Theology* (2019), pp. 400–433, but also in his *The Contradictory Christ* (Oxford: Oxford University Press, forthcoming).

[3] E.g., Thomas V. Morris, *The Logic of God Incarnate* (Ithaca: Cornell University Press, 1986); Thomas Senor, "Drawing on Many Traditions: An Ecumenical Kenotic Christology," in Anna Marmadoro and Jonathan Hill, eds., *The Metaphysics of the Incarnation* (Oxford: Oxford University Press, 2011), pp. 88–113; Stephen T. Davis, *Christian Philosophical Theology* (Oxford: Oxford University Press, 2006), pp. 172–192; Marilyn McCord Adams, *Christ and Horrors: The Coherence of Christology* (Cambridge: Cambridge University Press, 2006); Eleonore Stump, *Aquinas* (New York: Routledge, 2003), pp. 407–426; Brian Leftow, "The Humanity of God," in Anna Marmadoro and Jonathan Hill, eds., *The Metaphysics of the Incarnation* (Oxford: Oxford University Press, 2011), pp. 20–44; Oliver D. Crisp, "Compositional Christology Without Nestorianism," in Anna Marmadoro and Jonathan Hill, eds., *The Metaphysics of the Incarnation* (Oxford: Oxford University Press, 2011), pp. 45–66; Thomas P. Flint, "Should Concretists Part with Mereological Models of the Incarnation?" in Anna Marmadoro and Jonathan Hill, eds., *The Metaphysics of the Incarnation* (Oxford: Oxford University Press, 2011), pp. 67–87; Timothy Pawl, *In Defense of Conciliar Christology: A Philosophical Essay* (Oxford: Oxford University Press, 2016); Timothy Pawl, *In Defense of Extended Conciliar Christology: A Philosophical Essay* (Oxford: Oxford University Press, 2019).

Analytic Christology and the Theological Interpretation of the New Testament. Thomas H. McCall, Oxford University Press (2021). © Thomas H. McCall. DOI: 10.1093/oso/9780198857495.003.0007

without further explanation, that the historical Jesus of Nazareth was also God is as devoid of meaning as to say that this circle drawn with a pencil on paper is also a square."[4] Analytic philosophers of religion and theologians have risen to challenges such as that raised by Hick, and different proposals have been developed (or retrieved from the tradition) and defended against objections. We now have various combinations of metaphysics and doctrine: we have two-minds proposals with either abstractist or concretist metaphysics, we have both abstractist and concretist kenotic accounts on offer, we have "Model A's" and "Model T's." But for all the creativity and variety, what such proposals share in common is the commitment to demonstrate that Chalcedonian or, a bit more broadly, "conciliar" Christology is *not* contradictory. In other words, these proposals seek to show that there is no logical contradiction between the admittedly striking affirmations made by the creeds—and thus the Christology of the creeds should not be rejected on the grounds that it is necessarily false.

Beall takes a different approach. Indeed, it is a *very* different approach: he defends "the viability of 'Contradictory Christology'" by arguing that "the right response to the fundamental problem of Christology (viz., Christ's having two apparently complementary—contradiction-entailing—natures) is to accept the familiar contradictions."[5] Beall's fascinating proposal offers an important option for thinking about the doctrine of the incarnation. He makes this proposal with verve, clarity, and rigor, and his proposal raises some fascinating and important issues. In what follows, I first introduce his proposal and make a few observations about the role of logic in theology. I then mention for further consideration several issues that are raised by reflection on some of the historical and systematic theological considerations; I raise these not as lethal criticisms but as observations about the complications that would come with Beall's proposal. Following this, I focus on the reasoning patterns that are discernible in both the Pauline statements about Jesus Christ and in the statements of Jesus himself. I then make the case that, depending on how these statements are understood, they are either the basis of an important objection to Beall's proposal or, alternatively, the basis of a helpful support for one of his central theses.

[4] John Hick, "Jesus and the World Religions," in John Hick, ed., *The Myth of God Incarnate* (London: SCM Press, 1977), p. 178.
[5] Jc Beall, "Christ—A Contradiction: A Defense of a Contradictory Christology," *Journal of Analytic Theology* (2019), p. 401.

6.2 Divine and Human: The Proposal

Beall is convinced that the Chalcedonian statement gets Christology fundamentally correct; it is part of the true Christology. But he avers that most
defenders of conciliar Christology have erred in arguing that the doctrine as
such does not express a contradiction. The error, as he sees it, does not
concern the theological commitments but instead has to do with the underlying logic with which the defenders have worked to defend the doctrine. In
place of the older and flawed logic with which they were saddled, Beall
proposes the employment of paraconsistent logic.

6.2.1 Beall's Paraconsistent Logic

Just what is this logic? While a full account is far beyond the limits of this
discussion, it might be helpful to follow Beall's summary of the relevant
aspects.[6]

Beall takes the proper account of logical consequence to be absence of
counterexample. A "counterexample is a 'case' in which all the premises are
true but the conclusion is not true."[7] A relation of logical consequence is "an
absence-of-counterexample relation: a pair of sentences $A \therefore B$ (or, generally,
a pair from a set X to sentence B) is *logically valid* iff logic(-al consequence)
sees no counterexample to the pair, where a counterexample is a possibility
in which A (or everything in set X) is true but B fails to be true."[8]

Beall's account is what he refers to as *First Degree Entailment* (FDE).
A brief comparison of FDE with both "classical logic" (CL) and the "logic of
paradox" (LP) may help to illuminate the key features. CL demands both
completeness and consistency. As Beall puts it, "in any (classical) case, every
sentence is either true or false, and no sentence is both true and false."[9] LP
requires completeness but allows that some sentences may not be consistent;
every sentence must be true or false—but some sentences can be both true
and false.[10] FDE differs from both LP and CL, for FDE denies that a sentence
must be either complete or consistent. Some sentences are true; others are

---

[6] See also Chapter Two of Beall, *The Contradictory Christ*.

[7] Jc Beall and Shay Allen Logan, *Logic: The Basics*, second edition (New York: Routledge,
2017), p. 9.

[8] Jc Beall, "On Contradictory Christology: Preliminary Remarks, Notation and Terminology,"
Journal of Analytic Theology (2019), p. 437.

[9] Beall and Logan, *Logic*, p. 177.   [10] E.g., Beall and Logan, *Logic*, pp. 178, 194.

false. But other sentences are neither true nor false, and still others are both true and false.[11]

Beall asks us to "begin with the idea that there are two fundamental 'truth values,' The True and The False. Intuitively, the two values yield four 'possibilities' for any truth-bearer A: A is True; A is False; A is Both; and A is Neither (true nor false)."[12] CL demands both exhaustion (every sentence is either true or false) and exclusion (for no sentences are both true and false). LP requires exhaustion but not exclusion. But neither exclusion nor exhaustion are required for FDE.[13] CL does not allow for either "gaps" (in truth value, where something is neither true nor false) or "gluts" (an overdetermination of truth value, according to which something is both true and false). LP excludes gaps but not gluts. FDE allows for both gluts and gaps.

Beall's FDE is thus a version of dialetheism, "the view that some truths have true negations."[14] Beall observes that this "view has struck many philosophers as being both terribly radical and wholly implausible."[15] Surely Beall is correct in this assessment, and it is not hard to see reasons for this. Commitment to the "Law of Non-Contradiction" (LNC)—roughly, that "nothing is both true and false"—has been and remains strong.[16] One such reason is this: allowing a contradiction into our theory, or accepting a contradiction, confronts an "Explosion" into absurdity. The basic concern is that the acceptance of any true contradiction entails the acceptance of everything—and thus the acceptance of every contradiction. This objection to contradictions has been around for a very long time, and traditionally it has been expressed as *ex contradictione quodlibet*.[17]

---

[11] For completeness, I should note that Beall also discusses the so-called "Kleene" or K3 logical theory, which demands consistency but not completeness. See the discussion in Beall and Logan, *Logic*, e.g., pp. 178, 194.
[12] Jc Beall, "True and False—As If," in Graham Priest, Jc Beall, and Bradley Armour-Garb, eds., *The Law of Non-Contradiction: New Philosophical Essays* (Oxford: Oxford University Press, 2004), p. 198.
[13] Beall and Logan, *Logic*, pp. 202–204, 209, 242.   [14] Beall, "True and False," p. 197.
[15] Beall, "True and False," p. 197.
[16] Graham Priest, "What Is So Bad About Contradictions?" *Journal of Philosophy* (1998), p. 416. Some may object to reference to "the" law; Patrick Grim distinguishes between "at least four Laws of Non-Contradiction," "What Is A Contradiction?" in Graham Priest, Jc Beall, and Bradley Armour-Garb, eds., *The Law of Non-Contradiction: New Philosophical Essays* (Oxford: Oxford University Press, 2004), p. 55.
[17] Graham Priest traces it back to medieval logic (notably including John Duns Scotus), "What Is So Bad About Contradictions?" in Graham Priest, Jc Beall, and Bradley Armour-Garb, eds., *The Law of Non-Contradiction: New Philosophical Essays* (Oxford: Oxford University Press, 2004), pp. 24–25.

Greg Restall observes that the claim is less than immediately obvious; "commitment to a contradiction does not seem to compel rationally (or even to make rationally *more plausible*) commitment to absolutely everything whatsoever."[18] Accordingly, it might help to briefly sketch the argument for Explosion. As Beall (following C. I. Lewis) explains it, the gist of the argument goes like this:

(1) Assume that $A \wedge \sim A$ is true;
(2) By (1) and Simplification, A is true;
(3) By (2) and Addition, $A \vee B$ is true;
(4) By (1) and Simplification, $\sim A$ is true;
(5) But, then, by (3), (4), and Disjunctive Syllogism, B is true.[19]

Beall's FDE affirms Simplification and Addition, so rejection of (2), (3), and (4) is not an option. The response of the FDE defender will be to reject Disjunctive Syllogism—after all, the FDE-theorist might point out, the only reason to hold to Disjunctive Syllogism is a commitment to LNC. Without LNC, there is no affirmation of Disjunctive Syllogism—and without Disjunctive Syllogism, there is no threat of explosion.

The philosophical debates over LNC are ongoing and do not admit of easy resolution. Indeed, some philosophers judge them to be at an impasse. David Lewis, for example, thinks that the debate "instantly reaches dead-lock" and ends in a "complete stalemate."[20] Similarly, Patrick Grim concludes that "on some approaches" the defenders of LNC can gain a "victory [that] is easy but trivial," while on other approaches one can score an "easy but cheap victory for dialetheism."[21] With respect to Beall, however, we should be clear about two points: first, he is convinced that explosion does not follow as a strictly logical consequence; and, second, he maintains that explosion can be a real danger for theory-specific cases. For while "contradictions are not explosive according to logic" and thus "need not be

---

[18] Greg Restall, "Laws of Non-Contradiction, Laws of Excluded Middle, and Logics," in Graham Priest, Jc Beall, and Bradley Armour-Garb, eds., *The Law of Non-Contradiction: New Philosophical Essays* (Oxford: Oxford University Press, 2004), p. 77.

[19] Jc Beall, "Introduction: At the Intersection of Truth and Falsity," in Graham Priest, Jc Beall, and Bradley Armour-Garb, eds., *The Law of Non-Contradiction: New Philosophical Essays* (Oxford: Oxford University Press, 2004), pp. 5–6. See further the discussion in Aladdin M. Yaqub, *An Introduction to Logical Theory* (Buffalo: Broadview Press, 2013), p. 358.

[20] David Lewis, "Letters to Beall and Priest," in Graham Priest, Jc Beall, and Bradley Armour-Garb, eds., *The Law of Non-Contradiction: New Philosophical Essays* (Oxford: Oxford University Press, 2004), pp. 176–177.

[21] Grim, "What Is A Contradiction?", p. 58.

explosive in all true theories," nonetheless they "may be explosive in some" theories and in fact *are* explosive in many domains (e.g., mathematics, biology).[22] Indeed, Beall relies upon what he calls "the default consistency assumption," the assumption that "classical logic is perfectly reliable *in most cases*."[23] True contradictory theories are rare indeed.[24]

Even if the worries about explosion are successfully defused, however, we are left with Beall's own conclusion that "the following are *not* FDE-valid: excluded middle, non-contradiction, modus ponens, modus tollens" and "disjunctive syllogism."[25] In other words, according to Beall, none of the given patterns are *logically* valid (i.e., valid according to FDE); however, some or even all of these patterns can be—indeed are, according to Beall—valid according to theory-specific consequences.

6.2.2   Logic and Theology: An Appreciative Interlude

Before moving forward, I want, as a theologian, to state my hearty agreement with much of what Beall says about the role of logic in theology. He notes that any theory (in whatever field of inquiry) will include the (initial) truths that are basic to the theory and that motivate that theory. But any theory that strives for completeness and adequacy will also include "*whatever follows from the truths in the theory*; it should contain all of the *consequences* of a theory's claims."[26] Logic sorts out these relations of consequence; it helps us see what does—and what does not—follow from the first-order truth claims of the theory itself. I welcome much of what Beall says here, for logic has an important role to play in theology. As John Wesley—who is somewhat more renowned as an evangelist than a logician—puts it, logic is "necessary next to, and in order to, the knowledge of Scripture."[27] Despite the fact that it was considered "unfashionable" among the clergy of his time, nonetheless logic is invaluable. For with it we have the possibility of "apprehending things clearly, judging truly, and reasoning conclusively."[28] Logic "is good for this at least (wherever it is

---

[22] Beall, "Preliminary Remarks," p. 437.   [23] Beall, "True and False," p. 213.
[24] See further Beall, *The Contradictory Christ*, 1.4.
[25] Beall and Allen, *Logic*, p. 198. Cf. Beall, "True and False," p. 199.
[26] Beall, "Christ—A Contradiction," p. 403.
[27] John Wesley, "Address to the Clergy," in *The Works of John Wesley, Volume X: Letters, Essays, Dialogs, and Addresses* (Grand Rapids: Zondervan, n.d), p. 483.
[28] Wesley, "Address to the Clergy," p. 483.

understood), to make people talk less; by showing them both what is, and what is not, to the point; and how extremely hard it is to prove anything."[29]

Beall insists that "theology is no different" from other disciplines in this respect.[30] Logic is rightly said to be "'universal' and 'topic-neutral,'" and thus it includes theology.[31] I could not agree more. Systematic theology is ultimately about God, but it is also about all else as that "all else" relates to God.[32] As such, it includes not only core claims about God and the world but also whatever is entailed by those core claims. Thus "theologians must not only add various basic truths about God but also 'complete' (as far as possible) the theory via a consequence relation."[33] Accordingly, theologians should include in their theories not only those truths that they take to be revealed by God but also what truths of theological relevance really follow from those revealed truths. They should recognize that the entailments of what they affirm are also included in their doctrinal proposals.

This may seem obvious, but I am grateful for Beall's insistence here, and I hope that theologians will be properly appreciative of this point. For in modern and contemporary theology (in sharp contrast to much theology in the Christian tradition) it is sometimes too easy to find theologians making claims about the "implications" of some doctrinal proposal—either positively or negatively—without doing the hard work of seeing just what *is* implied or entailed. In other words, it is not uncommon to see theologians rush to celebrate the (desired) "implications" of some pet doctrinal proposal—but without pausing to demonstrate that the desired conclusions indeed are implied or entailed. Similarly, it is not hard to find theologians make affirmations and then deny the (undesired) implications; it is almost as if the operative assumption is that there are no such consequences if we do not *want* those consequences. A theologian may affirm some tenet of classical orthodoxy and then also affirm some other propositions that would entail the contradiction of that tenet—but then insist that there is no problem because they do not intend to affirm the contradictory proposition. But it is one thing to affirm some proposition A and deny some proposition B. It is another thing entirely to affirm some proposition A and deny some proposition B while also affirming some proposition C—when C entails the denial of A and/or the affirmation of B.[34]

---

[29] Wesley, "Address to the Clergy," p. 492.

[30] Beall, "Christ—A Contradiction," p. 404.

[31] Beall, "Christ—A Contradiction," p. 405.

[32] Cf. John B. Webster, "Principles of Systematic Theology," *International Journal of Systematic Theology* 11:1 (2009), pp. 56–71.

[33] Beall, "Christ—A Contradiction," p. 404.

[34] As Keith E. Yandell and I argue in "On Trinitarian Subordinationism," *Philosophia Christi* (2009), p. 357.

Beall concludes that "without a consequence (closure) relation our theories remain inadequate; they fail to contain truths that are entailed by the given set of truths. Inasmuch as theorists, and theologians in particular, aim to give as complete a theory of the target phenomenon as possible, the reliance on a consequence relation for our theory is required."[35] Beall is right that any theological theory should include whatever is entailed by the given set of truths. Amen—logic has an important role to play in theology, and theologians would do well to recognize this. As someone important in theology once said, "Come, let us reason together" (Isaiah 1:18).

But just what, more precisely, is the role of logic? Beall is unmistakably clear that it helps us trace consequences. But what does this mean, and does it do more? Logic (at least as it is standardly understood) is invaluable in demonstrating what follows from a proposition (and that proposition's conjunction with other propositions), what comes "downstream" of a set of claims, what comes as an entailment whether we want it or not. But is this all that it can do? Or can it make more substantive contributions to theology? More directly to the issue at hand, logic can show where contradiction follows as a consequence. But does logic also show us that those contradictions are *false only*—does it show that they are false only simply in virtue of being contradictions? Here we see with clarity how Beall's view takes leave of classical logic—on Beall's account, logic itself does not show that contradictions are false only. Various contradictions may in fact be false only, and indeed Beall is insistent that they should not be accepted widely in theology. But logic itself does not rule out contradictions, and it leaves open the door to the possibility that some may in fact be true (and, indeed, one contradiction—the set of claims contained in orthodox Christology—*is* true).

With this brief account of the relevant developments in logic at hand, we come to his doctrinal proposal.

6.2.3 The Christological Proposal

With this background sketch of Beall's logic, his Christological proposal is fairly straightforward: the apparent contradictions that are built into orthodox Christology are in fact genuine contradictions. They are to be affirmed as real contradictions, and the orthodox doctrine as formulated in the major

---

[35] Beall, "Christ—A Contradiction," p. 404.

THE LOGOS AND HIS LOGIC   185

creeds and conciliar statements is to be accepted and believed as such by
Christians. Christ is said to be both impassible and one who suffered, both
omniscient and limited in understanding and knowledge, both eternal and
temporally located. "The contradiction of Christ, on the proposed
Christology, is not there because the Conciliar-text authors were sloppy;
it's there because Christ's foundational role in Christianity requires something contradictory—and thereby something extraordinary, unique, and
awesome."[36]

6.3 The True and the False: Issues for Further Consideration

With this bit of background in mind, and with the core features of Beall's
proposal before us, we can proceed toward evaluation of his account. Here
are some issues that deserve further attention as analytic theologians think
about the appropriateness and usefulness of his approach.

6.3.1 Christ and His Creed

So what are we make of the apparent contradictions in the creeds and
conciliar statements? Beall notes that Timothy Pawl makes the case that it
is "at best uncharitable to interpret the conciliar fathers as advancing
anything close to a genuinely contradictory Christology."[37] On Pawl's
account (and I think that we could extend this beyond Pawl to other analytic
apostles of Christian orthodoxy), it would be uncharitable to do so because
this would mean that the conciliar fathers were asserting things that cannot
even possibly be true.[38] So, for the sake of charity, we should interpret them
as making claims about *apparent* contradictions. Beall disagrees. In fact, he
charges Pawl with an uncharitable reading because Pawl's account has the
conciliar fathers using the "key predicates in non-standard and undefined
ways."[39] So both Pawl and Beall want to promote a charitable reading.
Neither, so far as I can see, wants to read the creedal statements in such a

---

[36] Beall, "Christ—A Contradiction," p. 416.
[37] Beall, "Christ—A Contradiction," p. 420.
[38] Timothy J. Pawl, *In Defense of Conciliar Christology: A Philosophical Essay* (Oxford: Oxford University Press, 2016), pp. 84–85.
[39] Beall, "Christ—A Contradiction," p. 420.

way that implies that the conciliar fathers were simply incoherent, and neither wants a reading that is implausible. Thus Pawl assumes that they were not asserting something they took to be a genuine contradiction, and thus Beall assumes that they really meant to affirm the contradictions (since they just asserted them without making the sophisticated "Pawline" moves or watering them down). Both want a charitable reading. But they disagree about what that *is*.

Here are some observations. First, I take it that the creedal statements were intended neither, on the one hand, as mere "grammatical rules" or "linguistic regulation" (with no metaphysical commitments or constraints whatsoever), nor, on the other hand, as more-or-less complete explanations of the incarnation.[40] To interpret the creeds as either attempting full explanation or merely playing grammar-Nazi is, in my view, both uncharitable and quite implausible. I think that it is much better to think of the creedal statements as both making central affirmations ("here is what we *must* hold") and crucial denials ("here is what we *can't* believe")—and then leaving interpretive space for various possibilities and metaphysical development between the core of what we must hold and the boundaries beyond which we cannot go. If I am correct, then we should not expect them to make explicit their metaphysical and logical commitments as part of the creeds (or even as addendums).

Second, it seems to me that the any charitable reading will be one that allows for the possibility of coherence while not being historically implausible. So if we have reason to think that the framers and defenders of the conciliar statements were thinking along the lines of Beall's subclassical proposal, then interpreting them as making claims that they knew were directly contradictory might be the charitable way to go. But in the absence of such reasons, it becomes less plausible. And, if less plausible, then it is also less charitable, for then we are interpreting them as making overt contradictions—while also believing contradictions to be false.

So do we have such reasons? Commenting on the philosophical history, Nicholas Rescher and Robert Brandom note that "Since Aristotle's day, virtually all logicians and logically concerned philosophers in the mainstream Western tradition have had a phobia of inconsistency. They have been near to unanimous in proscribing it from the precincts of their logical

---

[40] The phrase "linguistic regulation" is taken from Sarah Coakley, "What Chalcedon Solved and Didn't Solve," in Stephen T. Davis, Daniel Kendall, S.J., and Gerald O'Collins, S.J., eds., *The Incarnation* (Oxford: Oxford University Press, 2002), pp. 143–163.

and ontological theorizing, holding that the toleration of inconsistencies would inevitably bring cognitive disaster in its wake."[41] This may be true of the philosophical history, but, not surprisingly, it is also true of the theological history. As Ephraim Radner points out, "Almost all the Fathers were wary of affirming that Scripture had within itself real 'contradictions,' a charge associated with the enemies of Scripture. And much effort was made to explain the presence of such *apparent* tensions within the texts."[42] What they took to be true about claims made within the text of Scripture they also took to be true more broadly.[43] With direct reference to Chalcedon, Coakley concurs:

> In a broadly accepted sense, the Chalcedonian "Definition" does indeed involve a "paradoxical" claim—the claim that "God" and "man," normally perceived as strikingly different in defining characteristics, find in Christ a unique intersection. Here "paradox" simply means "contrary to expectation," and the mind is led on from there to eke out an explanation that can satisfy both logic and tradition. However, we should be careful to distinguish this meaning of "paradox" from a tighter one in which not merely something "contrary to expectation" is suggested, but something self-contradictory... The overwhelming impression from following the debate leading up to Chalcedon, however, as well as that which succeeds it, is that the "paradoxical" nature of the incarnation in the first sense is embraced (with greater or lesser degrees of enthusiasm), but that "paradox" in the latter sense is vigorously warded off.[44]

If this is right (and I think that it is), then the efforts of Pawl (and his fellow apostles) should be seen as a kind of "eking out" effort. Pawl's is not the first such effort, and indeed it has a great deal of both formal and material continuity with important theologians within the Christian tradition. As such, it is neither uncharitable nor implausible.

Beall responds, however, by saying that the central issue is not historical but conceptual and systematic. The most important question is not "What

---

[41] Nicholas Rescher and Robert Brandom, *The Logic of Inconsistency: A Study of Non-Standard Possible-World Semantics and Ontology* American Philosophical Quarterly (Totowa, NJ: Rowan and Littlefield, 1979), p. 1.
[42] Ephraim Radner, *Time and the Word: Figural Readings of the Christian Scriptures* (Grand Rapids: William B. Eerdmans Publishing Co., 2016), p. 218.
[43] Gregory of Nyssa, *Against Eunomius*, 1.42.
[44] Coakley, "What Chalcedon Solved and Didn't Solve," pp. 154–155.

did the conciliar theologians who framed Chalcedon believe about logic?" Instead, the question we should be asking is: "What *should* they have thought about logic?" As he says, "The pressing question, to my mind, is not whether many theologians and philosophers are under the grip of the standard account of logic (-al consequences); the important question is whether they ought to be. Why hold that account?"[45] As Beall sees things, "a central part of charity aims for truth over what may've been fallacious intentions—based on erroneous beliefs—of the authors," and he concludes that a "charitable reading, on this view, can go against the intentions of the text's authors."[46]

It is interesting to consider what might have happened if the theologians of the fourth and fifth centuries who framed the statements of the ecumenical creeds had made use of Beall's account of logic. In other words, what would have happened if they had done what they "should" have done? The answer to that question is far from clear. It is less than obvious that we would have the very creedal statements that Beall takes to be expressing the true Christology. For without the pressure of the quest for logical consistency, we might not have the creeds—well, at least *these* creeds—at all. Consider the following scenario: in the mid-fifth century, a group of theologians and bishops are wrestling with the dictates of the earlier, received councils and the pressures brought to bear by the various aspects of the biblical witness to the person of Jesus Christ.[47] These theologians are faced with three major options. On one hand, they are presented with (what we now know as) the Chalcedonian Formula (what Beall takes to be part of the true Christology). But on the other hand, they are offered a precise creedal statement of Nestorian Christology. And there is more: on yet a third hand, they are given a monophysite statement that is consistent with the Council of Ephesus (431) but not with the Chalcedonian Formula.

Faced with these options, how are our bishops and theologians to respond? If they were to accept Beall's account of logic and opt for a Contradictory Christology, why should they choose one of these three options over the others? On what basis would they do so? Once we admit that Christ is a contradiction and thus that statements about him can be both true and false (when taken, of course, in the same sense), then why

[45] Beall, "Reply to McCall," p. 493.　　[46] Beall, "Reply to McCall," p. 493.

[47] Here I am deeply and gratefully indebted to Fr. Philip-Neri Reese for his questions to Jc and our subsequent discussion (during a workshop held on Contradictory Christology at the Center for Philosophy of Religion of the University of Notre Dame in February 2020).

would they conclude that Chalcedon gives the proper statement? Perhaps the answer is this: Chalcedon is correct precisely *because* it embraces the contradictory elements without attempting a resolution. But, again, why Chalcedon? What makes Chalcedon special in this respect? Chalcedon insists on one person who subsists in two natures. It rejects the view that Christ is two persons, and it likewise rules out any teaching according to which there is only one nature. But why be so restrictive? If we are going to allow contradictions as true, then why not simply say that it is true that Christ is exactly one person and also say that it is true that Christ is exactly two persons? Why not affirm both exactly one nature and exactly two natures (but not three)? Why not multiply the contradictions and make everyone happy?

If we accept contradictions as true, then it is not clear why we should not accept lots of contradictions as true. Even if we limit the true contradictions to the realm of Christology, we are still left to wonder why we should not accept many contradictions in Christology. More pointedly, we do not have reason to rule out the various heterodox views that are rejected by Chalcedon. If the pro-Nicene and pro-Chalcedonian theologians had known and accepted Beall's logic, would we even have Chalcedon (or even Nicaea)—and thus the "true Christology?" It is not at all obvious that we would.

6.3.2 Christ and His (Possible) Worlds

I take Beall's proposal to be one that is expressly logical rather than meta-physical in nature (although certainly not anti-metaphysical). As such, it would underdetermine the metaphysics and instead would allow for a range of metaphysical options. Beall intends for his account to be metaphysically neutral.[48] This is not to say that it would allow for just *any* metaphysics, and it may be the case that the logic will rule out some options in metaphysics. But which? And what will this mean for Christology?

In an earlier exchange, I raised this concern. More precisely, I asked how Beall's proposal maps onto issues of modality. Issues of modality are important in theology generally and in Christology specifically, and it is

---

[48] See Beall, *The Contradictory Christ*, 3.3.

not clear how Beall's proposal impacts our understanding of modality. One way of approaching this issue is to consider the following proposition

(T) *it is possible that there is at least one true contradiction.*

It seems obvious that Beall is committed to (T). Now compare it with

(NT) *it is not possible that there is at least one true contradiction.*

Now consider further the conjunction of (T) and (NT). Putting them together yields

(TNT) *it is possible that there is at least one true contradiction and it is not possible that there is at least one true contradiction.*

It seems obvious that (TNT) is not only *about* contradictions, (TNT) itself *is* a contradiction. But is (TNT) a true contradiction? Or does it suffer the inconvenience of being a false (and not-true) contradiction?

Suppose that (TNT) is true. If (TNT) is one of the true contradictions, then we are left to conclude not only that there is at least one true contradiction *and* that there are no true contradictions, we are also to conclude that what is possible is also impossible and even that what is necessary is also impossible. So what is true is also false, and what is *necessarily* false is also true. According to S5, $\Diamond p \Rightarrow \Box\Diamond p$. Thus the first conjunct of (TNT) cannot fail to be true if it is true at all. To put it in possible worlds semantics, if it is true at all, then it is true in all possible worlds.[49] Accordingly, there is at least one possible world where a contradiction is true, and it is true in all possible worlds that there is at least one possible world where a contradiction is true. But the second conjunct, if true, is also necessarily true (because $\sim\Diamond p = \Box\sim p$); it is true in all possible worlds. If the second conjunct is true, then there is no world in which the first conjunct is true; while if the first is true, then there is no world in which the second is true. Either way, there is no world in which both are true.

Initially, this raises at least two concerns. The first concerns intelligibility: it is not immediately obvious what it *means* to say that (TNT) is true. The

---

[49] Beall elsewhere endorses an understanding of necessity as truth in all possible worlds, e.g., Jc Beall and Greg Restall, *Logical Pluralism* (Oxford: Oxford University Press, 2006), p. 15.

second problem is that (TNT) would seem to give us modal collapse or maybe something even more worrisome (perhaps modal explosion). Where "modal collapse" happens when possibility is "collapsed" into necessity, here it seems we have the threat of *impossibility* collapsing into necessity, of necessary truth "collapsing" into necessary falsehood. Since I think that modality is important in theology (and that reality has a modal structure), I think that theology should be very wary of any theory with such consequences.

Suppose, on the other hand, that (TNT) is false. If (TNT) is false, then these consequences do not follow. So, it seems, the obvious thing to do is to reject (TNT) as false. But on what basis? The classical logician will immediately recognize that (TNT) is false and will reject it as such—(TNT) is not only about contradictions, it *is* a contradiction. Thus it is false. It is necessarily false, and not even Chuck Norris can make it true. There are a lot of hard problems in philosophy, but this is not one of them. End of story. But Beall's theory can hardly take this route. For on his view, as we have seen, logic is "clearly topic-neutral by not taking a stand on whether gappy or glutty sentences are ruled out."[50] With respect to some topics, it may indeed be the case that there is no room for gluttiness (with mathematics, this clearly *is* the case), while with respect to other matters, acceptance of gappiness and gluttiness may be appropriate. The salient point is that logic itself does not decide. As Beall puts it, subclassical "logic does not force unique, strange phenomena into the cramped confines of classical-logic possibilities" but "is silent on whether theorists *should* entertain a contradictory (glutty) theory." The upshot is that when considering the possibility of a true contradiction on the subclassical account, "logic itself, contrary to the standard account, doesn't rule it out."[51] Logic itself does not rule out (TNT). So if it is going to be eliminated, it will have to be on the basis of something theory-specific. However, in this case there is no other theory that (TNT) is about, and because there is no theory there are no theory-specific eliminators. It seems as though the contradiction in question is straightforwardly and merely about logic—modal logic—so we have neither logic itself nor other theory-specific criteria to guide us. If logic itself does not rule out the possibility of a true contradiction, then logic does not rule out this one. But neither is it obvious that anything else does (since this appears to be a logic-only matter).

[50] Beall, "Christ—A Contradiction," p. 414.
[51] Beall, "Christ—A Contradiction," p. 414.

So what are we to do with (TNT)? Rejecting the second conjunct outright seems to be against the grain of Beall's preferred subclassical account (committed, as it is, to inclusion of classical logic even as it expands around and beyond it). And to reject (TNT) as one of the false contradictions seems arbitrary (because logic itself cannot rule it out, and, as a logical matter, there is no theory-specific evidence that would do so). I guess we could say "so much the worse for thinking about modality." But perhaps instead we should conclude "so much the worse for any system that makes it so difficult to reject something so obviously problematic." But without good reason to reject either conjunct—and Beall's account is committed to the first and without obvious reason to reject the second (since, again, it would appear that the logic itself is neutral on the issue and we don't see any theory-specific reasons to reject it)—we are unsure how to avoid it. So taking (TNT) as true threatens modal collapse or explosion. Either way, should be worried about modal instability.

More broadly—and more importantly—we are left to wonder about the relationship between subclassical logic (as applied to theological issues) and modality. It is understandable that Beall does not address all such matters here; his is, after all, an essay on Christology rather than an essay on the relationship of subclassical logic to modal logic. But neither is this irrelevant, for modal considerations are important in theology. This is true generally, and Christology is no exception. Beall's account assumes that

> Christ has a divine nature (entailing immutability) and *independently and without diminishment* also has a human nature (entailing mutability).

This follows from orthodox Christology, but of course there is more to say. To the issue at hand, it is important to note that Christ has a divine nature *necessarily* but has a human nature *contingently*.[52] Theology needs an account of modality adequate to handle such affirmations.

Perhaps there are also good reasons for the subclassical logician to consider (TNT) to be one of the false contradictions and to reject it as such (in this case, one can think of my worries merely as potentially common misunderstandings that are likely to be made by theologians). Or perhaps it is the case that acceptance of subclassical logic will entail different

---

[52] See Richard Cross, *The Metaphysics of the Incarnation: Thomas Aquinas to Duns Scotus* (Oxford: Oxford University Press, 2002), p. 179.

understandings of modality.[53] If so, then it would be good to know the price; theologians should look carefully and count the cost before embracing it. I am confident that Beall has more to say about these matters. But accounting for modality in subclassical logic is not, as Beall elsewhere recognizes, "entirely straightforward."[54]

Or so I argued in the earlier engagement. In his thoughtful and helpful response, Beall observes that my "second horn involves the assumption that the so-called modal logic is logic."[55] There is a problem with this assumption; the problem is the "assumption that what's true of logic (-al consequence) is true of modal logic."[56] Beall makes a case that what is usually called "modal logic" really is not logic, strictly speaking, as much as it is metaphysics. Logic is all about consequence relations, and sometimes conceptual tools that pass themselves off as "logic" (e.g., Boolean logic) are actually "tributaries off the main stream of logic" but not exactly logic "in the important narrow sense" in Beall's preferred usage.[57] Beall does not wish to get into a war of words over the terminology itself, but he says that "so-called modal logic is so called not because it's logic (in the target, much narrower sense involved in debates over whether logical consequence is subclassical); it's so called because it's an account of the formal consequence relation underwriting our true theory of the given modal notions."[58] Logic "itself (i.e., logical consequence, not the extra-logical consequence relation involved in the true theory of modality)," Beall notes, "will not decide the issue."[59]

Fair enough. I take Beall's point: when talking about modal logic, we are really doing metaphysics rather than logic per se.[60] Accordingly, the horns of

[53]   Susan Haack sees modal logics (such as T, S4, and S5) as "supplements" to classical logic rather than "rivals" to it, *Deviant Logic: Some Philosophical Issues* (Cambridge: Cambridge University Press, 1974), p. 2. Jc Beall, Michael Glanzberg, and David Ripley note that "when they were first studied and understood," modal logics "were taken to be alternatives to classical logic; nowadays they are more commonly considered *extensions* of classical logic, retaining what was there but adding additional vocabulary." Jc Beall, Michael Glanzberg, and David Ripley, *Formal Theories of Truth* (Oxford: Oxford University Press, 2018), p. 39. On the other hand, Jc Beall and Bas C. van Frassen argue that "at some level at least we cannot think of modal logic as simply adding to or extending standard logic" (which they seem to equate with "classical propositional logic"), J. C. Beall and Bas C. van Frassen, *Possibilities and Paradox: An Introduction to Modal and Many-Valued Logic* (Oxford: Oxford University Press, 2003), p. 7.
[54]   Jc. Beall, "Truth, Necessity, and Abnormal Worlds," in M. Pelis, ed., *Logica Yearbook 2009* (College Publications, 2010), p. 11.
[55]   Beall, "Reply to McCall," p. 503.   [56]   Beall, "Reply to McCall," p. 503.
[57]   Jc Beall and Greg Restall, *Logical Pluralism* (Oxford: Oxford University Press, 2006), p. 8.
[58]   Beall, "Reply to McCall," p. 504.   [59]   Beall, "Reply to McCall," p. 504.
[60]   I say "may be right" because it is still less than obvious to me that it is so easy to separate the metaphysics of modality from the correct account of logic. Consider: when Beall gives the correct account of logical consequence, he says that it is the absence of counterexample, and he

what Beall calls "McCall's dilemma" are not sharp at all, and they do not imperil his account. However, we are left with the worrisome question: just how does Beall's proposal map on to issues of modality? Beall admits that "the true account of modality might well involve some fairly far-out 'worlds' where things behave wildly differently from the S5-like setting in the background of McCall's discussion."[61] Beall is not, to be sure, committed to the notion that the proper account of modality indeed *does have* such "wildly far-out elements," but he allows that it might.[62] He also says that "the development of Contradictory Christology must be explicit about the details of theologically relevant modal notions."[63] And so this is where we are left: we know that the metaphysics of modality are important for Christology (and, indeed, for the Contradictory version of it). But we are not quite sure what the proper account of it is. If it turns out that Contradictory Christology rules out S5, then that is a steep price to pay. So there is yet work to be done, and it is work that should be done before Contradictory Christology is embraced.

6.3.3 Christ and His Church

In my earlier exchange with Beall's proposal, I raised a question that is more directly practical and even pastoral in nature. This is a concern about the potential reception of Beall's proposal, which is, of course something over which Beall does not have much control. Nevertheless, given the argument he makes and the enthusiasm for affirming contradictions that one some-times finds among contemporary theologians who are not as careful as Beall, there are reasons for concern. The question is this: how is the account drawn here to offer helpful practical guidance for Christian communities if it is affirmed and applied more broadly? Nicholas Wolterstorff observes that

---

goes on to say that a counterexample is a "*possibility* in which A (or everything in set X) is true but B fails to be true," "Preliminary Remarks," p. 437 (emphasis mine). Similarly, Beall and Restall say that "Leibniz's vision of necessity as truth in all possible worlds is compelling," *Logical Pluralism*, p. 15. But once we are talking about possibility and necessity, then surely we are back in the realm of modality. And, when we are back in the realm of modality we are also talking about ontology and metaphysics. For further discussion of some of the complications arising at the intersection of modality and ontology, see Bob Hale, *Necessary Beings: An Essay on Ontology, Modality, and the Relations Between Them* (Oxford: Oxford University Press, 2013), pp. 103–110.

[61] Beall, "Reply to McCall," p. 502.   [62] Beall, "Reply to McCall," p. 502.

[63] Beall, "Reply to McCall," p. 503 n12.

theologians often have an urge to "heal the world."[64] More broadly, theology is (at least partially—there are debates over this) a *churchly* enterprise. Doctrine plays important roles in the formation of the community of faith and in the formation of character and the virtues within that faith community.[65] More particularly, Christology plays a determinative role not only in Christian doctrine but in Christian ethics. Will the acceptance of contradictions (in this case of the doctrine of the incarnation, at the very heart of the Christian faith, but potentially more broadly as well) actually strengthen the faith of the faithful and assist ecclesial communities in the important work in moral and spiritual formation? Or might it bring harm? Consider the following scenario.

The Pope and his Council of Cardinals, along with the Orthodox Patriarchs and Metropolitans, the Archbishop of Canterbury, and the relevant Protestant ecclesial leaders, embark on an ecumenical study of the debates over the ordination of women to the priesthood. They assemble the "ideal" team of scholars; they get the best theologians (of the various disciplines) gathered from the respective ecclesial groups. Notably, all parties agree that this is an ideal team. They lock themselves in the basement of the Vatican with the full range of resources. In other words, this is the All-Star team, they have all that they need, and they have as long as they need.

Something interesting and unexpected happens. The longer they are together, the more they become convinced that there are unassailable theological arguments for the restriction of ordination (to some set of ecclesial offices) to males—*and* they become increasingly convinced that there are unassailable theological arguments for opening ordination (to the full set of ecclesial offices) to women. Interestingly, both the "traditionalists" and the "progressives" are in substantial agreement on both accounts: scholars from both sides see and affirm the strength of the arguments for both conclusions. They seem to be stuck, and—because they tacitly assume that a contradiction cannot be true—they keep going back to the arguments. But each time they do so, they are even more deeply convinced of the theological case to be made for both conclusions.

---

[64] Nicholas Wolterstorff, "To Theologians: From One Who Cares About Theology but Is Not One of You," *Theological Education* (2005), p. 83.

[65] On this point see Ellen T. Charry, *By the Renewing of Your Minds: The Pastoral Function of Christian Doctrine* (Oxford: Oxford University Press, 1997).

Fortunately, however, the basement of the Vatican has decent internet access, and at some point a bishop who is frustrated by the situation seeks diversionary relief by reading the *Journal of Analytic Theology*. There he comes across a brilliant article commending "Contradictory Christology," and he is immediately taken by the idea that subclassical logic is appropriate for theology. The next morning he makes the case that it is appropriate for the issue before them; he argues that the only thing holding them up is this dang relic called the "Law of Non-Contradiction." What we need, he says, is a "glutty" theology of ordained ministry. The scholars and clerics agree. In one accord, this ideal team of ecumenical scholars issues an important statement: they conclude that the ordination of women to the priesthood is both theologically permissible and morally obligatory *and* that the ordination of women to the priesthood is both theologically impermissible and a grave sin. Understanding that this might be initially confusing to the catholic faithful, they include in their statement not only their strongest arguments for both views but also a short primer on subclassical logic.

The catholic faithful find this statement and accompanying explanations interesting but also super confusing. Indeed, they are frustrated by it, and they keep asking this question: "But what do we *do*?" They begin to hope that their leaders do not make similar progress on other contested issues. For while these sorts of exercises might be good for ecumenism considered abstractly, they are not good at all for the life and health of the church.

Christian theology attempts to tell the truth—the whole truth so far as we can—about God and all things as these are related to God. As the truth, it is supposed to shape and mold our characters (individually and communally), it is supposed to form us spiritually and morally, it is supposed to give us moral guidance. How can it do so if it includes contradictions (or even allows for their possibility)? Perhaps the answer is that there will be no true contradictions on matters with practical import; maybe it is the case that anytime there is a contradiction with respect to a practical, pastoral, or moral issue that itself is a clue that there must be some theory-specific reason to judge the contradiction false. Maybe so, but such a criterion might threaten to rule out the very Christological move being made by Beall.

Responding to this concern, Beall notes that "one question raised by McCall's scenario is whether it's possible."[66] "Clearly," he responds, "the

---

[66] Beall, "Reply to McCall," p. 505. See further the discussion in Beall, *The Contradictory Christ*, 4.5.

scenario is logically possible."[67] Beall also points out that to say this much is not to say a lot. Surely Beall is correct; possibilities come rather cheaply. Beall goes on to say that such a scenario is "at least implausible."[68] Again, Beall is correct. Such a scenario is, it is safe to say, *highly* implausible. Indeed, to say that it is highly implausible is a rather drastic understatement. Nonetheless, it remains a possibility, and it is also the case that the incarnation itself is highly implausible. Beall also allows that it may be relevant to the Vatican-basement case study to admit that "it's physically (or cognitively or the like) impossible... to both accept and simultaneously reject the truth of some claim *A*."[69] Indeed, but it also seems that such impossibility is also relevant for the claims of Contradictory Christology.

If contradictions are not believable, then it is hard to see how the claims of Contradictory Christology are to be believed. If they are believable, on the other hand, then I am concerned that claims of them will spread among theologians. Beall rightly anticipates a "very common reaction" to his proposal.[70] He wants to make it clear that he is *not* "proposing that theologians should seek to find contradictions willy nilly"; he is not suggesting "that theologians ought to seek out contradictions."[71] There is good reason, he insists, for us to reject most logical contradictions as false. True contradictions are very rare, for many are ruled out by the objects of inquiry themselves. His proposal, again, is that it is only on state occasions—notably, for our purposes, the incarnation—that the truth might require a genuine contradiction. He does not want to completely "rule out" the possibility that there may be other true contradictions in theology, but he clearly does not intend for this to be taken as license.[72]

Beall's own preferences are clear enough, but I am not sanguine about their reception among theologians. I worry that many theologians will indeed take what Beall says as open season on the constraints of classical logic and, more importantly, to license contradictions galore.[73] It is not hard to imagine a theologian being convinced by Beall and then saying, "Cool, I no

---

[67] Beall, "Reply to McCall," p. 505.   [68] Beall, "Reply to McCall," p. 506.

[69] Beall, "Reply to McCall," p. 506.   [70] Beall, "Christ—A Contradiction," p. 416.

[71] Beall, "Christ—A Contradiction," p. 416. Recall Beall's commitment to the "Default Consistency Assumption," "True and False," p. 213.

[72] Beall, "Christ—A Contradiction," p. 422.

[73] Ephraim Radner discusses several recent theologians (most notably Pavel Florensky and Vladimir Lossky) who make explicit and positive use of contradiction, and he references the work of Graham Priest. See the discussion in *Time and the Word*, pp. 216–219. See further Pavel Florensky, *The Pillar and Ground of Truth: An Orthodox Theodicy in Twelve Letters*, trans. Boris Jakim (Princeton: Princeton University Press, 1997), pp. 106–123.

longer need to worry about avoiding contradictions." Beall might remonstrate with "No, you theologians should not 'seek out contradictions.'"[74] But the theologian's response is quick: "look, we don't have to seek them out—they are all over the place and come looking for us. They are unavoidable. The good news now is that we don't need to worry about them."

My worry, in other words, is that contemporary theologians might take Beall seriously—too seriously. Beall says that "until there's good reason to accept that our true theories of phenomena beyond Christ are likewise glutty I see no reason not to reject the spread of contradictory theories."[75] But a theologian converted to Beall's position may wonder what reasons there might be not to *accept* the spread of such theories. Contradictions will be seen as delightfully if perhaps recklessly mischievous—but will become dangerously promiscuous. Not only will logic in theology be "gappy" (where the "law of excluded middle" is rejected and the proposition may be neither true nor false) and "glutty" (where the "law of contradiction" is rejected and the proposition may be both true and false), it will also be overly promiscuous.

Beall responds by insisting that "theology is plainly contradictory at just one core point—the incarnation."[76] He wants to make his own position "clearer than crystal: there may be true contradictions beyond the core contradiction who is Christ; but a giddy quest for making Christianity contradictory at every whim is not only (to use McCall's term) promiscuous; it is simply silly, irresponsible 'theorizing' which, pending a good reason to think otherwise, would appear to me to not be after truth at all."[77] Beall indeed has succeeded in this respect; he has made his own views "clearer than crystal." I am not, however, as sanguine as he seems to be. I want to know: what are the good reasons to avoid licensing the spread of contradictions in theology? Indeed, could it be that there are distinctly *theological* reasons?

6.4 The Lord's Logic

Recall Beall's admission that "the following are *not* FDE-valid: excluded middle, non-contradiction, modus ponens, modus tollens" and "disjunctive syllogism."[78]

---

[74] Beall, "Christ—A Contradiction," p. 416.
[75] Beall, "Christ—A Contradiction," p. 419.   [76] Beall, "Reply to McCall," p. 495.
[77] Beall, "Reply to McCall," p. 495.
[78] Beall and Logan, *Logic*, p. 198. Cf. Beall, "True and False," p. 199.

6.4.1 Dominical Counterexamples?

Some philosophers and theologians have pointed to what appears to be the use such non-FDE-valid forms of argument in the biblical witness to Christ. Dallas Willard, for instance, refers to "Jesus the Logician." He clarifies what he means by this appellation:

> Now when we speak of "Jesus the logician" we do not, of course, mean that he developed theories of logic, as did, for example, Aristotle and Frege. No doubt he could have, if he is who Christians have taken him to be. He could have provided a *Begriffsschrift*, or a *Principia Mathematica*, or alternative axiomatizations of Modal Logic, or various completeness or incompleteness proofs for various "languages" ... He could have. Just as he could have handed Peter or John the formulas of Relativity Physics or the Plate Tectonic theory of the earth's crust, etc.... But he did not do it, and for reasons which are bound to seem pretty obvious to anyone who stops to think about it. But that, in any case, is not my subject here. When I speak of "Jesus the logician" I refer to his *use* of logical insights: to his mastery and employment of logical principles in his work as a teacher and public figure.[79]

Willard offers additional clarifications: Jesus is not using logic to hammer people with arguments but to win them over, and Jesus's arguments are sometimes understated and enthymematic. But, for Willard, it is obvious that Jesus used logic in his parables and stories as well as his sermons and pronouncements. And, for Willard, it is also plain that Jesus used the "two primary logical relations" of "implication (logical entailment) and contradiction" and thus licenses use of "standard forms of argument such as the Barbara Syllogism, Disjunctive Syllogism, Modus Ponens and Modus Tollens ... "[80]

Consider some (purported) examples. Willard illustrates Jesus's employment of logic by pointing to passages that tell of Jesus's interpretation of ritual law (Matt 12:1-8); here Willard says that while Jesus is focused upon the distinctly *theological* and *moral* considerations (rather than as a lesson in logic), he does so by approaching these issues "in terms of the logical inconsistency of those who claim to practice it [the law] in the manner

---

[79] Dallas Willard, "Jesus the Logician," *Christian Scholars Review* XXVIII:4 (1999), pp. 605–606.
[80] Willard, "Jesus the Logician," p. 606.

officially prescribed at the time."[81] Similarly, Willard shows how Jesus defeats the attempted *reductio* that was brought against him by the Sadducees (Luke 20:27-40), and he draws upon Jesus's own employment of a *reductio* in his "obviously self-conscious use of logic" (Luke 20:40-43; cf. Matt 5:29-30). Other theologians and philosophers find other texts to illustrate Jesus's employment of logic. For instance, Norman L. Geisler and Patrick Zuckeran conclude that Jesus is making use of Disjunctive Syllogism (Matt 6:24; 12:30; Luke 11:23; 16:13) when he demands complete allegiance. As they put it, "Since Jesus claims to be God, there is no neutral position. For either he is accepted as God and obeyed, or he is not accepted as God and not obeyed. And if one does not obey God, then he is opposed to God."[82]

When Paul reflects on the central Christian affirmations, he also appears to make use of argumentative forms common to classical logic. In his first letter to the Corinthians, he says

> Now if Christ is proclaimed as raised from the dead, how can some of you say that there is no resurrection from the dead? If there is no resurrection of the dead, Christ has not been raised, and if Christ has not been raised, then our proclamation has been in vain and your faith has been in vain. We are even found to be misrepresenting God, because we testified of God that he raised Christ—whom he did not raise if it is true that the dead are not raised. For if the dead are not raised, then Christ has not been raised. If Christ has not been raised, your faith is futile and you are still in your sins. Then those also who have died in Christ have perished. If for this life only we have hoped in Christ, we are of all people most to be pitied.

> But in fact Christ has been raised from the dead, the first fruits of those who have died. For since death came through a human being, the resurrection of the dead has also come through a human being; for as all die in Adam, so all will be made alive in Christ.   (1 Cor 15:12-22)

Paul's teaching here is dense and compact, and clearly there is plenty to digest. For our purposes, however, we can see that it is not implausible to read Paul's sermon as someone who is making an argument using Modus Ponens, Modus Tollens, and the tools of classical logic more generally.

---

[81]   Willard, "Jesus the Logician," p. 608.
[82]   Norman L. Geisler and Patrick Zukeran, *The Apologetics of Jesus: A Caring Approach to Dealing with Doubters* (Grand Rapids; Baker Books, 2009), p. 72.

It seems plausible that Paul is responding to a modus ponens type of argument that is commonly known among the Corinthians. He says "if there is no resurrection from the dead, then Christ has not been raised..." (1 Cor 15:13), and the argument to which he is responding might be summarized as:

(6) If there are no resurrections, then Christ has not been resurrected;[83]
(7) There are no resurrections;
(8) Therefore, Christ has not been resurrected.

Taken this way, Paul responds with a modus tollens argument:

(6)   If there are no resurrections, then Christ has not been resurrected;
(9)   Christ has been resurrected (see 15:4-8);
(10) Therefore, it is not the case that there are no resurrections.

There is, of course, a great deal more than this in Paul's message. But whatever exactly we are to make of the full sermon, it is clear that Paul insists—emphatically, without hesitation or qualification—that *Christ is risen from death*. He does not say that *Christ is risen from death* is true but also false. Nor, of course, does he say that *Christ is risen from death* is neither true nor false. To the contrary, he boldly proclaims *Christ is risen from death* as true. He proclaims it as unambiguously true, straightforwardly true. For Paul, *Christ is risen from death* is true and not-false. He does not entertain the notion that both *Christ has been resurrected* and *There are no resurrections* (or *resurrections are not possible*) are true. He takes it to be an analytic truth that *there are no resurrections* (or *resurrections are not possible*) is false if *Christ has been resurrected* is true.[84] Of course he is positive that Christ *has* been resurrected, so he is sure that *there are no resurrections* (and *resurrections are not possible)* is false. It is because of this conviction that Paul is also confident that faith is not useless, preaching is not pointless, that he is not guilty of bearing false witness against God, and that those who have died "in Christ" are not lost. So it looks like the tools of classical logic play an important role in Paul's proclamation of the gospel.

---

[83] Perhaps the argument is stronger and runs along the lines of

  (6*) If resurrections are impossible, then Christ has not been resurrected."
[84] Thanks to Rich Davis for helpful conversation here.

6.4.2 Christ and Contradiction

What might this mean for Beall's proposal? If Beall's account of FDE (and rejection of Disjunctive Syllogism, Modus Ponens, and Modus Tollens) is correct, does this mean that Paul and Jesus were committing logical errors of the most basic sort? Was Paul doing so not in talking about secondary, tertiary, or even trivial matters (if Paul *ever* talked about trivial matters, such as March Madness brackets or their first century equivalents) but instead when proclaiming the gospel? Worse yet, was Jesus—the one believed by Christians to be divine and thus omniscient—clueless about logical consequence? Or, on the other hand, is Paul's proclamation of the good news simply bad news for Beall's account of logic?

It seems to me that the most promising way for Beall to respond is this: accept the patterns of reasoning presented by Paul and Jesus as valid and appropriate but then say that "the validity of the pattern is not logical validity but rather some theory-specific validity relation turning on the theory's constraints on the given predicates."[85] An advantage of this response for Beall is that it is entirely consistent with what he (repeatedly) says elsewhere: on FDE, logic *alone* does not rule out contradictions or give us explosion, but in *many* (indeed, *most* or *almost all*) theories, it is not possible that contradictions are true and in point of fact contradictions do yield explosion. So even though there is nothing about logic itself that rules out contradictions, there are theory-specific cases aplenty that in fact *do* prohibit the possibility of true contradictions. The matters discussed in the aforementioned teachings of Jesus, and indeed his own resurrection from death, fall into this category. When it comes to resurrections, there are theory-specific prohibitions of the acceptance of contradictions. Thus there is nothing inconsistent here; the teachings of Jesus and the most important preaching of Paul do not present a counterexample to Beall's FDE account of logic.

---

[85] Jc Beall, "Three Ways of Detachment: Notes for Tom McCall," private correspondence, 8 February 2020. Beall offers two additional ways of responding to the challenge I've presented here (which he takes very seriously). One way is to tie material detachment (cf., positively and forwardly, Modus Ponens, or negatively and backwardly, Modus Tollens) to a binary accessibility relation and then account for the material detachment as $A \Rightarrow B$ as referring to a case in which "at possibility x there's no x-accessible point y such that A is true at y but B untrue at y." The other way is simply to consider this an instance of "acceptance and rejection behavior," according to which the general way to proceed is to think that "gluts are few and far between" and that "we generally reject !A as an option, and simply infer B from both A and $A \Rightarrow B$" (where !A is Beall's shorthand for a contradiction $A \wedge \sim A$). I am deeply appreciative of Jc's willingness to discuss this further with me and for his generosity.

It is not a stretch to think that this sort of response will generate further questions. Philosophically, it might seem to be unacceptably ad hoc. For the strategy allows and even affirms contradictions with respect to the core elements of the doctrine (as creedally formulated, at least) but then resists and rejects them with respect to other vitally important elements of Christology (viz., resurrection). A defender of Beall's position will reject the charge of *ad hocness*, of course, insisting that we should always opt for the theory that is not only consistent but also simplest and *full*.[86] Since going for the "full theory" gives us the "recalcitrant data" that forces us to affirm the fundamental contradiction in the case of the person of Christ, then we in fact should affirm the contradiction. But since we can account for the resurrection-data without falling back to contradiction, then we should do exactly that.

Theologically, some may worry that this move separates the *person* of Christ from the *work* of Christ. When we consider the work of Christ, we do not—and arguably should not—accept contradictions. When we consider his teaching, we do not accept contradictories as true. When he says "Do not think that I have come to abolish the law or the prophets; I have not come to abolish but to fulfill" (Matt 5:17) we should not conclude that we both should and should not think that he has come to abolish or that we both should and should not think that he has come to fulfill. When he says "Do not resist an evildoer" (Matt 5:39) and "Love your enemies and pray for those who persecute you" (Matt 5:44), we should not conclude that what he meant was "love and hate" your enemies (Matt 5:43). When we read the apostolic witness to the work of Christ telling us that "Christ suffered for you, leaving you an example, so that you should follow in his steps" (1 Peter 2:21), we do not conclude that he both did and did not leave an example. When we read that the Son became incarnate "so that through death he might destroy the one who has the power of death, that is, the devil, and free those who all their lives were held in slavery by the fear of death" (Heb 2:14-15), we should not think that he both did and did not destroy the one who holds the power of death.[87] When we read that Christ "redeemed us from the curse of the law by becoming a curse for us" (Gal 3:13), we are not to conclude that he both did and did not redeem us from the curse of the law. But, as we can see in many of these texts, the ministry or work of Christ is

---

[86] See Chapter Six of *The Contradictory Christ*.

[87] "Did" and "did not" here refers to the same sense, of course. This is not to deny the important issues of eschatological inauguration and fulfillment.

linked very closely to the person of Christ. "Since, therefore, the children share flesh and blood, he himself likewise shared the same things, so that through death he might..." (Heb 2:14). It is difficult if not impossible to make sense of the work of Christ—his teaching, his example, his representative and substitutionary death, his victorious resurrection, glorious ascension, and regal session—if we allow contradictions *there*. But since his work is based upon his person and closely linked to it, it is also hard to accept the notion that all this work is based upon a fundamental contradiction. The strength of this concern will probably have a lot to do with the more precise understandings of the relation of Christ's person to his work, but this will likely be an issue for further consideration.

So where does this leave us? The teaching of Jesus and the preaching of Paul appear to offer counterexamples to Beall's FDE-reliant proposal of Contradictory Christology. But appearances can be deceiving, and Beall can respond by saying that, with respect to such proclamation, the patterns of reasoning are theory-specific and thus do not serve as counterexamples. The extent to which such a response will allay concerns will surely be the subject of ongoing discussion. Taking Beall's way out would leave us with a very odd conclusion: with respect to the teachings of (Paul and) Jesus, while we would not exactly conclude that Jesus is saying "Do as I say, not as I do," we would be left with "Do as I say, not as *I Am*." But one thing should be abundantly clear: even if we accept the theory-specific way out for Beall's proposal, we are *not* licensed to accept contradictions willy-nilly in theology. If we do theology as we should, if we do theology by "going on in the same way" as Jesus and the apostles, then we should *not* either seek out or even accept claims of contradictions (beyond the fundamental contradiction at the heart of orthodox Christology).[88] Surely this should be good news for Beall's proposal of Contradictory Christology.

6.5 Conclusion

Jc Beall's proposal is a genuinely new and interesting development in Christology. It is bold and rigorous. It offers a novel way of accepting and

---

[88] Here I use the phrase (though not the full meaning) of Kevin Hector. See Kevin Hector, *Theology Without Metaphysics: God, Language, and the Spirit of Recognition* (Cambridge: Cambridge University Press, 2011), p. 38. For appreciative engagement and healthy critique, see Michael C. Rea, "Theology Without Idolatry or Violence," *Scottish Journal of Theology* (2011), pp. 61–79.

defending a venerable doctrine. It deserves careful philosophical and theological engagement.

In this chapter, I have attempted to offer a bit of that theological engagement—albeit in an "early" and perhaps impressionistic, rather piecemeal sense. Accordingly, I have raised several such areas that deserve further engagement. After first introducing the revolutionary proposal and the nonstandard, paraconsistent, philosophically "heterodox" logic undergirding it, I have centered attention on several theological issues. I have looked at creedal and traditional matters; here I raised issues related to proper interpretation of the creeds as well as considerations raised by attention to the history of the relevant debates and the development of Christological dogma. I then brought attention to several theologically important metaphysical (and especially modal) complications that seem to come with the paraconsistent approach. Following this, I turned attention to ecclesial and even pastoral concerns. Finally, I raised textually grounded issues related to the portrayals of the preaching of Paul and the teaching of Jesus himself in the New Testament.

Beall's radical proposal is a novel position on an old doctrine. It raises theologically (as well as philosophically) interesting issues. What it *does not do* is license theological contradictions more broadly.

Bibliography

Abraham, William J. "Systematic Theology as Analytic Theology," in Oliver D. Crisp and Michael C. Rea, eds., *Analytic Theology: New Essays in the Philosophy of Theology* (Oxford: Oxford University Press, 2009), pp. 54–69.

Adams, Marilyn McCord. *Christ and Horrors: The Coherence of Christology* (Cambridge: Cambridge University Press, 2006).

Adams, Marilyn McCord. *What Sort of Human Nature? Medieval Philosophy and the Systematics of Christology* (Milwaukee: Marquette University Press, 1999).

Allen, R. Michael. *The Christ's Faith: A Dogmatic Account* (New York: T&T Clark, 2009).

Allen, Richard. *The Life, Experience, and Gospel Labors of Rt. Rev. Richard Allen: To Which is Annexed the Rise and Progress of the African Methodist Episcopal Church in the United States of America, Containing a Narrative of the Yellow Fever in the Year of Our Lord 1793, with an Address to the People of Color in the United States* (Philadelphia: Ford and Ripley, 1880).

Alsted, Johannes-Heinrich. *Theologica Polemica* (Hanover, 1620).

Anatolios, Khaled. *Retrieving Nicaea: The Development and Meaning of Trinitarian Doctrine* (Grand Rapids: Baker Academic, 2011).

Aquinas, Thomas. *Summa Theologica*. Complete English Edition in Five Volumes, trans. the Fathers of the English Dominican Province (New York: Benzinger Bros., 1948).

Aquinas, Thomas. *Super Epistolam B. Pauli ad Hebraeos Lectura*, translated as *Commentary on the Letter of Saint Paul to the Hebrews*, trans. F. R. Larcher, eds. J. Mortensen and E. Alarcon (Lander, WY: The Aquinas Institute for the Study of Sacred Doctrine, 2012).

Attridge, Harold. *The Epistle to the Hebrews: A Commentary on the Epistle to the Hebrews*, Hermeneia (Philadelphia: Fortress Press, 1989).

Ayres, Lewis. "'As We Are One:' Thinking into the Mystery," in Oliver D. Crisp and Fred Sanders, eds., *Advancing Trinitarian Theology: Explorations in Constructive Dogmatics* (Grand Rapids: Zondervan Academic, 2014), pp. 94–113.

Baker, Lynne Rudder. "Making Sense of Ourselves: Self-Narratives and Personal Identity," *Phenomenology and the Cognitive Sciences* 15:1 (2016), pp. 7–15.

Barclay, John M. G. *Paul and the Gift* (Grand Rapids: William B. Eerdmans Publishing Co., 2015).

Barclay, John M. G. "Paul's Story: Theology as Testimony," in Bruce W. Longenecker, ed., *Narrative Dynamics in Paul: A Critical Assessment* (Louisville: Westminster John Knox Press, 2002), pp. 133–156.

Barth, Karl. *Church Dogmatics*, trans. G. W. Bromiley, eds., G. W. Bromiley and T. F. Torrance (Edinburgh: T&T Clark, 1956).

Bartholomew, Craig. "Listening for God's Address," in Craig G. Bartholomew and David J. H. Beldman, eds., *Hearing the Old Testament* (Grand Rapids: William B. Eerdmans Publishing Co., 2012).

Bauckham, Richard. *Gospel of Glory: Major Themes in Johannine Theology* (Grand Rapids: Baker Academic, 2015).

Bauckham, Richard. *Jesus and the God of Israel: God Crucified and Other Studies on the New Testament's Christology of Divine Identity* (Grand Rapids: William B. Eerdmans Publishing Co., 2009).

Bauckham, Richard. "Monotheism and Christology in the Gospel of John," in Richard N. Longenecker, ed., *Contours of Christology in the New Testament* (Grand Rapids: William B. Eerdmans Publishing Co., 2005), pp. 148–166.

Beall, Jc. "Christ – A Contradiction: A Defense of Contradictory Christology," *Journal of Analytic Theology* 7 (2019), pp. 400–433.

Beall, Jc. "Introduction: At the Intersection of Truth and Falsity," in Graham Priest, Jc Beall, and Bradley Armour-Garb, eds., *The Law of Non-Contradiction: New Philosophical Essays* (Oxford: Oxford University Press, 2004), pp. 1–19.

Beall, Jc. "On Contradictory Christology: Preliminary Remarks, Notation, and Terminology," *Journal of Analytic Theology* 7 (2019), pp. 434–439.

Beall, Jc. *The Contradictory Christ* (Oxford: Oxford University Press, forthcoming).

Beall, Jc. "Three Ways of Detachment: Notes for Tom McCall," private correspondence (8 February 2020).

Beall, Jc. "True and False – As If," in Graham Priest, Jc Beall, and Bradley Armour-Garb, eds., *The Law of Non-Contradiction: New Philosophical Essays* (Oxford: Oxford University Press, 2004), pp. 197–216.

Beall, Jc, Michael Glanzberg, and David Ripley. *Formal Theories of Truth* (Oxford: Oxford University Press, 2018).

Beall, Jc and Shay Allen Logan. *Logic: The Basics*, second edition (New York: Routledge, 2017).

Beall, Jc and Greg Restall. *Logical Pluralism* (Oxford: Oxford University Press, 2006).

Beall, Jc and Bas C. van Fraasen. *Possibilities and Paradox: An Introduction to Modal and Many-Valued Logic* (Oxford: Oxford University Press, 2003).

Bertschmann, D. H. "*Ex Nihilo* or *Tabula Rasa*? God's Grace between Freedom and Fidelity," *International Journal of Systematic Theology* 22:1 (2020), pp. 29–46.

Bickle, John. "Empirical Evidence for a Narrative Concept of Self," in Gary D. Fireman, Ted E. McVay, Jr., and Owen J. Flanagan, eds., *Narrative and Consciousness: Literature, Psychology, and the Brain* (Oxford: Oxford University Press, 2003), pp. 195–208.

Brower, Jeffrey E. and Michael C. Rea. "Material Constitution and the Trinity," *Faith and Philosophy* (2005), pp. 57–76.

Bruce, F. F. *The Epistle to the Hebrews*, revised edition, New International Commentary on the New Testament (Grand Rapids: William B. Eerdmans Publishing Co., 1990).

Brummer, Vincent. *The Model of Love: A Study in Philosophical Theology* (Cambridge: Cambridge University Press, 1993).

Brunner, Emil. *The Christian Doctrine of God, Dogmatics: Vol. 1*, trans. Olive Wyon (Philadelphia: Westminster Press, 1949).

Calvin, John. *The Epistle of Paul the Apostle to the Hebrews and the First and Second Epistles of St. Peter*, trans. William B. Johnson and eds. David W. Torrance and Thomas F. Torrance (print on demand).

Campbell, Douglas. *The Deliverance of God: An Apocalyptic Rereading of Justification in Paul* (Grand Rapids: William B. Eerdmans Publishing Co., 2009).

Campbell, Douglas. *Pauline Dogmatics* (Grand Rapids: William B. Eerdmans Publishing Co., 2020).

Campbell, Douglas A. *The Quest for Paul's Gospel: A Suggested Strategy* (New York: T&T Clark, 2005).

Campbell, Douglas A. "Romans 1:17 – A *Crux Interpretum* for the πίστις Χριστου Debate," *Journal of Biblical Literature* 113:2 (1994), pp. 265–285.

Carson, D. A. *The Gospel According to John* (Grand Rapids: William B. Eerdmans Publishing Co., 1991).

Casey, Paul M. *From Jewish Prophet to Gentile God: The Origins and Development of New Testament Christology* (Louisville: Westminster John Knox Press, 1991).

Charry, Ellen. *By the Renewing of Your Minds: The Pastoral Function of Christian Doctrine* (Oxford: Oxford University Press, 1997).

Chester, Stephen. "Apocalyptic Union: Martin Luther's Account of Faith in Christ," in Michael J. Thate, Kevin J. Vanhoozer, Constantine R. Campbell, eds., *"In Christ" in Paul: Explorations of Paul's Theology of Union and Participation* (Grand Rapids: William B. Eerdmans Publishing Co., 2018), pp. 375–398.

Christman, John. "Narrative Unity as a Condition of Personhood," *Metaphilosophy* 35:5 (2004), pp. 695–713.

Chrysostom, John. "Commentary on Galatians," in Philip Schaff ed., *A Select Library of the Nicene and Post-Nicene Fathers of the Christian Church*, Vol. XIII (Grand Rapids: William B. Eerdmans Publishing Co., 1994).

Coakley, Sarah. "What Chalcedon Solved and Didn't Solve," in Stephen T. Davis, Daniel Kendall, S. J., and Gerald O'Collins, S. J., eds., *The Incarnation* (Oxford: Oxford University Press, 2002), pp. 143–163.

Cockerill, Gareth Lee. *The Epistle to the Hebrews*, New International Commentary on the New Testament (Grand Rapids: William B. Eerdmans Publishing Co., 2012).

Crisp, Oliver D. "Analytic Theology as Systematic Theology," *Journal of Open Theology* 3:1 (2017), pp. 156–166.

Crisp, Oliver D. "Compositional Christology Without Nestorianism," in Anna Marmadoro and Jonathan Hill, eds., *The Metaphysics of the Incarnation* (Oxford: Oxford University Press, 2011), pp. 45–66.

Crisp, Oliver D. "On Analytic Theology," in Oliver D. Crisp and Michael C. Rea, eds., *Analytic Theology: New Essays in the Philosophy of Theology* (Oxford: Oxford University Press, 2009), pp. 33–53.

Cross, Richard. *Duns Scotus on God* (Aldershot: Ashgate, 2005).

Cross, Richard. *The Metaphysics of the Incarnation: Thomas Aquinas to Duns Scotus* (Oxford: Oxford University Press, 2002).

Das, A. Andrew. *Galatians* (St. Louis: Concordia Publishing House, 2014).

Davis, Stephen T. *Christian Philosophical Theology* (Oxford: Oxford University Press, 2006).

de Boer, Martinus C. *Galatians: A Commentary* (Louisville: Westminster John Knox Press, 2011).

Dempsey, Michael T., ed. *Trinity and Election in Contemporary Theology* (Grand Rapids: William B. Eerdmans Publishing Co., 2011).

DeSilva, David. *Perseverance in Gratitude: A Socio-Rhetorical Commentary on the Epistle "to the Hebrews"* (Grand Rapids: William B. Eerdmans Publishing Co., 2000).

Diller, Kevin. "Is God *Necessarily* Who God Is? Alternatives for the Trinity and Election Debate," *Scottish Journal of Theology* 66:2 (2013), pp. 209–220.

Duby, Steven J. *Divine Simplicity: A Dogmatic Account*, T&T Clark Studies in Systematic Theology (New York: Bloomsbury T&T Clark, 2016).

Dunn, James D. G. "Faith, Faithfulness," in *The New Interpreters Bible Dictionary Vol. 2: D-H* (Nashville: Abingdon Press, 2007), pp. 407–423.

Dunn, James D. G. "Once More, *ΠΙΣΤΙΣ ΧΡΙΣΤΟΥ*," reprinted in Richard Hays, *The Faith of Jesus Christ: The Narrative Substructure of Galatians 3:1–4:11*, second edition (Grand Rapids: William B. Eerdmans Publishing Co., 2002), pp. 714–744.

Dunn, James D. G. *Theology of Paul the Apostle* (Grand Rapids: William B. Eerdmans Publishing Co., 1998).

Dunn, James D. G. *The Theology of Paul's Letter to the Galatians* (Cambridge: Cambridge University Press, 1993).

Easter, Matthew C. "The *Pistis Christou* Debate: Main Arguments and Responses in Summary," *Currents in Biblical Research* 9:1 (2010), pp. 33–47.

Eastman, Susan G. *Paul and the Person: Reframing Paul's Anthropology* (Grand Rapids: William B. Eerdmans Publishing Co., 2017).

Eastman, Susan G. "The Shadow Side of Second-Person Engagement: Sin in Paul's Letter to the Romans," *European Journal of Philosophy of Religion* 5:4 (2013), pp. 125–144.

Eastman, Susan G. *Recovering Paul's Mother Tongue: Language and Theology in Galatians* (Grand Rapids: William B. Eerdmans Publishing Co., 2007).

Eastman, Susan G. "Knowing and Being Known: Interpersonal Cognition and the Knowledge of God," in Andrew B. Torrance and Thomas H. McCall, eds., *Knowing Creation: Perspectives from Theology, Philosophy, and Science* (Grand Rapids: Zondervan Academic, 2018), p. 157.

Elliott, Mark W. "*πίστις Χριστου* in the Church Fathers and Beyond," in Michael F. Bird and Preston M. Sprinkle, eds., *The Faith of Jesus Christ: Exegetical, Biblical, and Theological Studies* (Peabody: Hendrickson Publishers, 2009), pp. 277–289.

Ellis, Brannon. *Calvin, Classical Trinitarianism, and the Aseity of the Son* (Oxford: Oxford University Press, 2012).

Emery, Gilles. *The Trinitarian Theology of St Thomas Aquinas* (Oxford: Oxford University Press, 2007).

Emery, Gilles. "The Trinity," in Eleonore Stump and Brian Davies, eds., *The Oxford Handbook of Aquinas* (Oxford: Oxford University Press, 2012).

Evans, C. Stephen. *The Historical Christ and the Jesus of Faith: The Incarnational Narrative as History* (Oxford: Oxford University Press, 1996).

Fee, Gordon D. *Pauline Christology: An Exegetical-Theological Study* (Peabody: Hendrickson Publishers, 2007).

Feser, Edward. *Scholastic Metaphysics: A Contemporary Introduction* (Heusentamm: Editiones Scholasticae, 2014).

Flint, Thomas P. "Molinism and Incarnation," in Ken Perszyk, ed., *Molinism: The Contemporary Debate* (Oxford: Oxford University Press, 2011), pp. 187–207.

Flint, Thomas P. "Should Concretists Part with Mereological Models of the Incarnation?" in Anna Marmadoro and Jonathan Hill, eds., *The Metaphysics of the Incarnation* (Oxford: Oxford University Press, 2011), pp. 67–87.

Florensky, Pavel. *The Pillar and Ground of Truth: An Orthodox Theodicy in Twelve Letters*, trans. Boris Jakim (Princeton: Princeton University Press, 1997).

Forbes, William. *Considerationes Modestae et Pacificae Contoversiarum* (Oxford, 1850).

Forrest, Peter. "Divine Fission: A New Way of Moderating Social Trinitarianism," *Religious Studies* 34:2 (1998), pp. 281–297.

Freddoso, Alfred J. "Human Nature, Potency, and the Incarnation," *Faith and Philosophy* 3:1 (1986), pp. 27–53.

Freddoso, Alfred J. "Medieval Aristotelianism and the Case Against Secondary Causation in Nature," in Thomas V. Morris, ed., *Divine and Human Action: Essays in the Metaphysics of Theism* (Ithaca: Cornell University Press, 1988), pp. 74–118.

Friedeman, Caleb T., ed., *Listen, Understand, Obey: Essays on Hebrews in Honor of Gareth Lee Cockerill* (Eugene: Pickwick Publications, 2017).

Funk, Robert, Roy W. Hoover, and the Jesus Seminar. *The Five Gospels: The Search for the Authentic Words of Jesus* (New York: Macmillan Publishing Co., 1993).

Gallaher, Brandon. *Freedom and Necessity in Modern Trinitarian Theology* (Oxford: Oxford University Press, 2016).

Gathercole, Simon. *The Preexistent Son: Recovering the Christologies of Matthew, Mark, and Luke* (Grand Rapids: William B. Eerdmans Publishing Co., 2005).

Gaventa, Beverly Roberts. "The Singularity of the Gospel Revisited," in Mark W. Elliott, Scott J. Hafemann, N. T. Wright, and John Frederick, eds., *Galatians and Christian Theology: Justification, the Gospel, and Ethics in Paul's Letter* (Grand Rapids: Baker Academic, 2014), pp. 187–199.

Goldingay, John. "Biblical Narrative and Systematic Theology," in Joel B. Green and Max Turner, eds., *Between Two Horizons: Spanning New Testament Studies and Systematic Theology* (Grand Rapids: William B. Eerdmans Publishing Co., 2000), pp. 123–142.

Goldingay, John. *Do We Need the New Testament? Letting the Old Testament Speak for Itself* (Downers Grove: InterVarsity Academic, 2015).

Gorman, Michael J. *Inhabiting the Cruciform God: Kenosis, Justification, and Theosis in Paul's Narrative Soteriology* (Grand Rapids: William B. Eerdmans Publishing Co., 2009).

Gray, Patrick. *Godly Fear: The Epistle to Hebrews and the Greco-Roman Critiques of Superstition* (Atlanta: Society of Biblical Literature, 2003).

Grim, Patrick. "What Is A Contradiction?" in Graham Priest, Jc Beall, and Bradley Armour-Garb, eds., *The Law of Non-Contradiction: New Philosophical Essays* (Oxford: Oxford University Press, 2004), pp. 49–72.

Gunton, Colin. *The Promise of Trinitarian Theology* (Edinburgh: T&T Clark, 1991).

Haack, Susan. *Deviant Logic: Some Philosophical Issues* (Cambridge: Cambridge University Press, 1974).

Hale, Bob. *Necessary Beings: An Essay on Ontology, Modality, and the Relations Between Them* (Oxford: Oxford University Press, 2013).

Hampson, Daphne. *Christian Contradictions: The Structures of Lutheran and Catholic Thought* (Cambridge: Cambridge University Press, 2001).

Hampson, Daphne. "Luther on the Self: A Feminist Critique," *Word and World* 8:4 (1988), pp. 334–342.

Hampton, Stephen. *Anti-Arminians: The Anglican Reformed Tradition from Charles II to George I* (Oxford: Oxford University Press, 2008).

Hansen, Walter. *Galatians* (Downers Grove: InterVarsity Academic, 2010).

Hardy, Edward R., ed. *The Christology of the Later Fathers* (Louisville: Westminster John Knox Press, 1977).

Hasker, William. *Metaphysics and the Tri-Personal God*, Oxford Studies in Analytic Theology, eds., Michael C. Rea and Oliver D. Crisp (Oxford: Oxford University Press, 2013).

Hays, Richard. *Echoes of Scripture in the Letters of Paul* (New Haven: Yale University Press, 1989).

Hays, Richard. *The Faith of Jesus Christ: The Narrative Substructure of Galatians 3:1–4:11*, second edition (Grand Rapids: William B. Eerdmans Publishing Co., 2002).

Hector, Kevin. "God's Triunity and Self-Determination: A Conversation with Karl Barth, Bruce McCormack and Paul Molnar," *International Journal of Systematic Theology* 7:3 (2005).

Hector, Kevin. *Theology Without Metaphysics: God, Language, and the Spirit of Recognition* (Cambridge: Cambridge University Press, 2011).

Hick, John, ed. *The Myth of God Incarnate* (London: SCM Press, 1977).

Holmes, Stephen R. "Classical Trinity: Evangelical Perspective," in Jason Sexton, ed., *Two Views on the Doctrine of the Trinity* (Grand Rapids: Zondervan Academic, 2014), pp. 25–48.

Holmes, Stephen R. "Response to Thomas H. McCall," in Jason Sexton, ed., *Two Views on the Doctrine of the Trinity* (Grand Rapids: Zondervan Academic, 2014), p. 143.

Hooker, Morna D. "Another Look at πίστις Χριστου," *Scottish Journal of Theology* 69:1 (2016), pp. 46–62.

Hudson, Hud. "Fission, Freedom, and the Fall," in Jonathan Kvanvig, ed., *Oxford Studies in Philosophy of Religion* (Oxford: Oxford University Press, 2009), pp. 58–79.

Hughes, P. E. *Commentary on the Epistle to the Hebrews* (Grand Rapids: William B. Eerdmans Publishing Co., 1977).

Hunn, Debbie. "Debating the Faithfulness of Jesus Christ in Twentieth Century Scholarship," in Michael F. Bird and Preston M. Sprinkle, eds., *The Faith of Jesus Christ: Exegetical, Biblical, and Theological Studies* (Peabody: Hendrickson Publishers, 2009), pp. 23–33.

Hunsinger, George. "Election and the Trinity: Twenty-Five Theses on the Theology of Karl Barth," in Michael T. Dempsey, ed., *Trinity and Election in Contemporary Theology* (Grand Rapids: William B. Eerdmans Publishing Co., 2011), pp. 91–114.

Hunsinger, George. *How To Read Karl Barth: The Shape of His Theology* (Oxford: Oxford University Press, 1991).

Hunsinger, George. *Reading Barth with Charity: A Hermeneutical Proposal* (Grand Rapids: Baker Academic, 2015).

Hurd, Ryan M. "*Dei Via Regia:* The Westminster Divine Anthony Tuckney on the Necessity of Works for Salvation," *Westminster Theological Journal* 81:1 (2019), pp. 1–17.

Ingham, Mary Beth and Mechthild Dreyer. *The Philosophical Vision of John Duns Scotus* (Washington: The Catholic University of America Press, 2004).

Jamieson, R. B. *Jesus's Death and Heavenly Offering in Hebrews* (Cambridge: Cambridge University Press, 2019).

Jamieson, R. B. "When and Where Did Jesus Offer Himself? A Taxonomy of Recent Scholarship on Hebrews," *Currents in Biblical Research* 15:3 (2017), pp. 338–368.

Jipp, Joshua W. "Douglas Campbell's Apocalyptic, Rhetorical Paul: A Review Article," *Horizons in Biblical Theology* 32:2 (2010), pp. 183–197.

John of Damascus *De Fide Orthodoxa* III.11 *NPNF* 9.

Johnson, H. Wayne. "The Paradigm of Abraham in Galatians 3:6-9," *Trinity Journal* 8 (1987), pp. 179–199.

Johnson, Luke Timothy. *Hebrews: A Commentary* (Louisville: Westminster John Knox Press, 2006).

Johnson, Luke Timothy. "Romans 3:21-26 and the Faith of Jesus," *Catholic Biblical Quarterly* 44:1 (1982), pp. 77–90.

Jones, Paul Dafyyd. *The Humanity of Christ: Christology in Karl Barth's Church Dogmatics* (London: Continuum/T&T Clark, 2008).

Jones, Paul Dafyyd. "Obedience, Trinity, and Election: Thinking with and Beyond the *Church Dogmatics*," in Michael T. Dempsey, ed., *Trinity and Election in Contemporary Theology* (Grand Rapids: William B. Eerdmans Publishing Co., 2011), pp. 138–161.

Kaiser, Walter, Jr. *Recovering the Unity of the Bible: One Continuous Story, Plan, and Purpose* (Grand Rapids: Zondervan Academic, 2009).

Keating, Daniel. "Thomas Aquinas on the Epistle to the Hebrews: 'The Excellence of Christ,'" in Jon C. Laansma and Daniel J. Treier, eds., *Christology, Hermeneutics, and Hebrews: Profiles from the History of Interpretation* (New York: Bloomsbury T&T Clark, 2012), pp. 84–99.

Keck, Leander. "'Jesus' in Romans," *Journal of Biblical Literature* 108:3 (1989), pp. 443–460.

Kilby, Karen. "Projection and Perichoresis: Problems with Social Doctrines of the Trinity," *New Blackfriars* 81 (2000), pp. 432–445.

Kilby, Karen. "The Trinity and Politics: An Apophatic Approach," in Oliver D. Crisp and Fred Sanders, eds., *Advancing Trinitarian Theology: Explorations in Constructive Dogmatics* (Grand Rapids: Zondervan Academic, 2014), pp. 75–93.

Kostenberger, Andreas J. and Scott R. Swain. *Father, Son, and Holy Spirit: The Trinity and John's Gospel* (Downers Grove: InterVarsity Academic, 2008).

Kripke, Saul. *Naming and Necessity* (Cambridge, MA: Harvard University Press, 1972).

Lane, William L. *Word Biblical Commentary, Hebrews 1–8* (Nashville: Thomas Nelson, 1991).

Leftow, Brian. "Anti Social Trinitarianism," in Thomas McCall and Michael C. Rea, eds., *Philosophical and Theological Essays on the Trinity* (Oxford: Oxford University Press, 2009), pp. 52–88.

Leftow, Brian. "The Humanity of God," in Anna Marmadoro and Jonathan Hill, eds., *The Metaphysics of the Incarnation* (Oxford: Oxford University Press, 2011), pp. 20–44.

Leftow, Brian. "Modes Without Modalism," in Peter van Inwagen and Dean Zimmerman, eds., *Persons, Human and Divine* (Oxford: Oxford University Press, 2007), pp. 357–375.

Legge, Dominic, O. P. *The Trinitarian Christology of St Thomas Aquinas* (Oxford: Oxford University Press, 2017).

Lewis, David. "Letters to Beall and Priest," in Graham Priest, Jc Beall, and Bradley Armour-Garb, eds., *The Law of Non-Contradiction: New Philosophical Essays* (Oxford: Oxford University Press, 2004), pp. 176–177.

Lewis, David. *Philosophical Papers*, Vol. 1 (Oxford: Oxford University Press, 1983).

Linebaugh, Jonathan. "The Christo-centrism of Faith in Christ: Martin Luther's Reading of Galatians 2.16, 19-20," *New Testament Studies* (2013), pp. 535–544.

Linebaugh, Jonathan. "Incongruous and Creative Grace: Reading *Paul and the Gift* with Martin Luther," *International Journal of Systematic Theology* 22:1 (2020), pp. 47–59.

Linebaugh, Jonathan. "The Speech of the Dead: Identifying the No Longer and Now Living 'I' of Galatians 2:20," *New Testament Studies* 66:1 (2019), pp. 87–105.

Locke, John. *An Essay Concerning Human Understanding*, ed. P. Nidditch (Oxford: Oxford University Press, 1979).

Loke, Andrew. *The Origin of Divine Christology* (Cambridge: Cambridge University Press, 2017).

Lombard, Peter. *Sentences, Book Three: On the Incarnation of the Word*, trans. Guilio Silano (Toronto: Pontifical Institute of Medieval Studies, 2008).

Longenecker, Richard N. *Galatians*. Word Biblical Commentary 41 (Grand Rapids: Zondervan Academic, 1990).

Lowe, E. J. *A Survey of Metaphysics* (Oxford: Oxford University Press, 2002).

Macaskill, Grant. "Dynamic Reciprocity and Ontological Affinity in the Pauline Account of Solidarity," *International Journal of Systematic Theology* 22:1 (2020), pp. 18–28.

Macaskill, Grant. *Union with Christ in the New Testament* (Oxford: Oxford University Press, 2013).

Martyn, J. Louis. "World Without End or Twice-Invaded World," in Christine Roy Yoder, et al., eds., *Shaking Heaven and Earth: Essays in Honor of Walter Brueggeman and Charles B. Cousar* (Louisville: Westminster John Knox Press, 2005), pp. 117–132.

Matera, Frank J. *Galatians: A New Translation with Introduction and Commentary* (New York: Doubleday, 1997).

Matlock, Barry. "'Even the Demons Believe': Paul and πίστις Χριστου," *Catholic Biblical Quarterly* 64:2 (2002), pp. 300–318.

Matlock, R. Barry. "Zeal for Paul but Not According to Knowledge: Douglas Campbell's War on 'Justification Theory,'" *Journal for the Study of the New Testament* 34:2 (2011), pp. 115–149.

Matlock, Barry. "πίστις in Gal 3:26: Neglected Evidence for 'Faith in Christ?'" *New Testament Studies* 49:3 (2003), pp. 433–439.

McCall, Thomas H. *Forsaken: The Trinity and the Cross, and Why It Matters* (Downers Grove: InterVarsity Academic, 2012).

McCall, Thomas H. *An Invitation to Analytic Christian Theology* (Downers Grove: InterVarsity Academic, 2015).

McCall, Thomas H. "Gender and the Trinity Once More: A Review Article," *Trinity Journal* 36:2 (2015), pp. 263–280.

McCall, Thomas H. "Trinity Doctrine, Plain and Simple," in Oliver D. Crisp and Fred Sanders, eds., *Advancing Trinitarian Theology: Explorations in Constructive Dogmatic* (Grand Rapids: Zondervan Academic, 2014), pp. 42–59.

McCall, Thomas H. *Which Trinity? Whose Monotheism? Philosophical and Systematic Theologians on the Metaphysics of Trinitarian Theology* (Grand Rapids: William B. Eerdmans Publishing Co., 2010).

McCall, Thomas H. and Michael C. Rea, "Introduction," in Thomas H. McCall and Michael C. Rea, eds., *Philosophical and Theological Essays on the Trinity* (Oxford: Oxford University Press, 2009), pp. 1–15.

McCall, Thomas H. and Keith E. Yandell, "On Trinitarian Subordinationism," *Philosophia Christi* 11:2 (2009), pp. 339–358.

McCormack, Bruce L. "Election and the Trinity: Theses in Response to George Hunsinger," in Michael T. Dempsey, ed., *Trinity and Election in Contemporary Theology* (Grand Rapids: William B. Eerdmans Publishing Co., 2011), pp. 134–137.

McCormack, Bruce L. "Grace and Being: The Role of God's Gracious Election in Karl Barth's Theological Ontology," in John Webster, ed., *The Cambridge Companion to Karl Barth* (Cambridge: Cambridge University Press, 2000), pp. 92–110.

McCormack, Bruce L. "The Identity of the Son: Karl Barth's Exegesis of Hebrews 1.1-4 (and Similar Passages)," in Jon C. Laansma and Daniel J. Treier, eds., *Christology, Hermeneutics, and Hebrews: Profiles from the History of Interpretation* (New York: Bloomsbury T&T Clark, 2012), pp. 155–172.

McCormack, Bruce L. *Orthodox and Modern: Studies in the Theology of Karl Barth* (Grand Rapids: Baker Academic, 2008).

McCormack, Bruce L. "Seek God Where He May Be Found: A Response to Edwin Chr. van Driel," *Scottish Journal of Theology* 60:1 (2007), pp. 62–79.

McCormack, Bruce L. "With Loud Cries and Tears: The Humanity of the Son in the Epistle to the Hebrews," in Richard Bauckham, Daniel R. Driver, Trevor A. Hart, and Nathan MacDonald, eds., *The Epistle to the Hebrews and Christian Theology* (Grand Rapids: William B. Eerdmans Publishing Co., 2009), pp. 37–68.

McFarland, Ian. *In Adam's Fall: A Meditation on the Christian Doctrine of Original Sin* (Oxford: Wiley-Blackwell, 2010).

McFarland, Ian. *In Adam's Fall: A Meditation on the Christian Doctrine of Original Sin* (Oxford: Wiley-Blackwell, 2010).

Michael J. Loux, Michael J. "Introduction" to *The Possible and the Actual: Readings in the Metaphysics of Modality*, ed. Michael J. Loux (Ithaca: Cornell University Press, 1979), pp. 15–64.

Moffitt, David. *Atonement and the Logic of Resurrection in the Epistle to the Hebrews* (Leiden: Brill, 2013).

Moffitt, David. "It Is Not Finished: Jesus' Perpetual Atoning Work as the Heavenly High Priest in Hebrews," in Jon C. Laansma, George H. Guthrie, and Cynthia Long Westfall, eds., *So Great A Salvation: A Dialogue on the Atonement in Hebrew* (New York: Bloomsbury T&T Clark, 2019), pp. 157–175.

Molnar, Paul D. *Divine Freedom and the Immanent Trinity: In Dialogue with Karl Barth and Contemporary Theology* (Edinburgh: T&T Clark, 2002).

Molnar, Paul D. *Faith, Freedom and the Spirit: The Economic Trinity in Barth, Torrance, and Contemporary Theology* (Downers Grove: InterVarsity Academic, 2015).

Morris, Thomas V. *The Logic of God Incarnate* (Ithaca: Cornell University Press, 1986).

Muller, Richard A. *Dictionary of Latin and Greek Theological Terms, Drawn Principally from Protestant Scholastic Theology* (Grand Rapids: Baker Academic, 1985).

Muller, Richard A. *Post-Reformation Reformed Dogmatics: The Rise and Development of Reformed Orthodoxy, ca. 1520 to ca. 1725, Volume Four: The Triunity of God* (Grand Rapids: Baker Academic, 2003).

Muller, Richard A. *Post-Reformation Reformed Dogmatics: The Rise and Development of Reformed Orthodoxy, ca. 1520 to ca. 1725, Volume Three: The Divine Essence and Attributes* (Grand Rapids: Baker Academic, 2003).

Murray, Paul D. "Thomas Aquinas and the Potential Catholic Integration of a Dynamic Occasionalist Understanding of Grace," *International Journal of Systematic Theology* 22:1 (2020), pp. 83–112.

Maximus the Confessor. *On the Lord's Prayer PG* 90.

Nelson, Hilde Lindemann. *Damaged Identities, Narrative Repair* (Ithaca: Cornell University Press, 2001).

Nimmo, Paul T. "Barth and the Election-Trinity Debate: A Pneumatological View," in Michael T. Dempsey, ed., *Trinity and Election in Contemporary Theology* (Grand Rapids: William B. Eerdmans Publishing Co., 2011), pp. 162–181.

Noonan, Harold. *Personal Identity* (New York: Routledge, 1991).

Norman L. Geisler and Patrick Zukeran. *The Apologetics of Jesus: A Caring Approach to Dealing with Doubters* (Grand Rapids: Baker Books, 2009).

O'Brien, Peter. *The Letter to the Hebrews* Pillar New Testament Commentary (Grand Rapids: William B. Eerdmans Publishing Co., 2010).

Oderberg, David S. *Real Essentialism* (New York: Routledge, 2007).

Olson, Eric T. and Karsten Witt. "Narrative and Persistence," *Canadian Journal of Philosophy* 49:3 (2019), pp. 419–434.

Oord, Thomas Jay. "Can God Be Essentially Loving Without Being Essentially Social? An Affirmation of and Alternative for Keith Ward," *Philosophia Christi* 18:2 (2016), pp. 353–361.

Parfit, Derek. "Personal Identity," *Philosophical Review* 80:1 (1971), pp. 3–27.

Parfit, Derek. *Reasons and Persons* (Oxford: Oxford University Press, 1984).

Pawl, Timothy. *In Defense of Conciliar Christology* (Oxford: Oxford University Press, 2016).

Pawl, Timothy. *In Defense of Extended Conciliar Christology* (Oxford: Oxford University Press, 2018).

Peeler, Amy Beverage. "If Son, Then Priest," in Caleb T. Friedeman, ed., *Listen, Understand, Obey: Essays on Hebrews in Honor of Gareth Lee Cockerill* (Eugene: Pickwick Publications, 2017), pp. 95–115.

Peeler, Amy Beverage. *You Are My Son: The Family of God in the Epistle to the Hebrews* (New York: Bloomsbury T&T Clark, 2014).

Perry, John. "The Importance of Being Identical," in A. Rorty, ed., *The Identities of Persons* (Berkeley: University of California Press, 1976), pp. 67–90.

Pierce, Madison. *Divine Discourse in the Epistle to the Hebrews: The Recontextualization of Spoken Quotations of Scripture* (Cambridge: Cambridge University Press, 2020).

Piscator, Johannes. *Analysis Logica Sex Epistolarum Pauli, editio secunda* (n.p., 1593).

Plantinga, Alvin. "Essence and Essentialism," in Jaegwon Kim and Ernest Sosa, eds., *A Companion to Metaphysics* (Oxford: Blackwell, 1995), pp. 138–140.

Plantinga, Alvin. *The Nature of Necessity* (Oxford: Oxford University Press, 1974).

Plantinga, Alvin. *Warranted Christian Belief* (Oxford: Oxford University Press, 2000).

Plantinga, Cornelius, Jr. "Social Trinity and Tritheism," in Ronald J. Feenstra and Cornelius Plantinga, Jr., eds., *Trinity, Incarnation, and Atonement: Philosophical and Theological Essays* (Notre Dame: University of Notre Dame Press, 1989), pp. 21–47.

Plantinga, Cornelius, Jr. "The Threeness/Oneness Problem and the Trinity," *Calvin Theological Journal* 23:1 (1988), pp. 37–53.

Polanus, Amandus. *Collegium Anti-Bellarminianum* (Basel, 1613).

Porter, Stanley E. and A. W. Pitts. "πίστις with an Preposition and Genitive Modifier: Lexical, Semantic, and Syntactic Considerations in the πίστις Χριστου Discussion," in Michael F. Bird and Preston M. Sprinkle, eds., *The Faith of Jesus Christ: Exegetical, Biblical, and Theological Studies* (Peabody: Hendrickson Publishers, 2009), pp. 33–56.

Priest, Graham. "What Is So Bad About Contradictions?" *Journal of Philosophy* 95:8 (1998), pp. 410–426.

Priest, Graham, Koji Tanaka and Zach Weber. "Paraconsistent Logic," in Edward Zalta, ed., *Stanford Encyclopedia of Philosophy*, <https://plato.stanford.edu/arch ives/win2012/entries/davidson/>.

Pruss, Alexander R. and Joshua L. Rasmussen. *Necessary Existence* (Oxford: Oxford University Press, 2018).

Radde-Gallwitz, Andrew. *Basil of Caesarea, Gregory of Nyssa, and the Transformation of Divine Simplicity* (Oxford: Oxford University Press, 2009).

Radner, Ephraim. *Time and the Word: Figural Readings of the Christian Scriptures* (Grand Rapids: William B. Eerdmans Publishing Co., 2016).

Rahner, Karl. *The Trinity* (New York: Crossroad, 1997).

Rea, Michael C. "Introduction," in Oliver D. Crisp and Michael C. Rea, eds., *Analytic Theology: New Essays on the Philosophy of Theology* (Oxford: Oxford University Press, 2009), pp. 1–30.

Rea, Michael C. "Relative Identity and the Doctrine of the Trinity," in Thomas McCall and Michael C. Rea, eds., *Philosophical and Theological Essays on the Trinity* (Oxford: Oxford University Press, 2009), pp. 249–262.

Rea, Michael C. "Theology Without Idolatry or Violence," *Scottish Journal of Theology* 68:1 (2011), pp. 61–79.

Rea, Michael C. "The Metaphysics of Original Sin," in Peter van Inwagen and Dean Zimmerman, eds., *Persons: Human and Divine* (Oxford: Oxford University Press, 2007), pp. 319–356.

Rea, Michael C. and Jeffrey E. Brower. "Material Constitution and the Trinity," in Thomas McCall and Michael C. Rea, eds., *Philosophical and Theological Essays on the Trinity* (Oxford: Oxford University Press, 2009), pp. 263–282.

Rescher, Nicholas and Robert Brandom. *The Logic of Inconsistency: A Study of Non-Standard Possible-World Semantics and Ontology* American Philosophical Quarterly (Totowa, NJ: Rowan and Littlefield, 1979).

Restall, Greg. "Laws of Non-Contradiction, Laws of Excluded Middle, and Logics," in Graham Priest, Jc Beall, and Bradley Armour-Garb, eds., *The Law of Non-Contradiction: New Philosophical Essays* (Oxford: Oxford University Press, 2004), pp. 73–84.

Richard of St. Victor. *De Trinitate PL* 196.

Richard of St. Victor. *Trinity and Creation*, Victorine Texts in Translation: Exegesis, Theology, and Spirituality from the Abbey of St. Victor, Boyd Taylor Coolman and Dale M. Coulter, eds. (New York: New City Press, 2011).

Rowe, C. Kavin. "Luke and the Trinity: An Essay in Ecclesial Biblical Theology," *Scottish Journal of Theology* 56:1 (2003), pp. 1–26.

Rutherford, Samuel. *Examen Arminianismi* (Utrecht, 1668).

Rutherford, Samuel. *A Survey of the Spirituall Antichrist* (London, 1648).

Schectman, Marya. *The Constitution of Selves* (Ithaca: Cornell University Press, 1996).

Schectman, Marya. "Empathic Access: The Missing Ingredient in Personal Identity," *Philosophical Explorations* 4:2 (2001), pp. 95–111.

Schreiner, Thomas R. Schreiner, *Hebrews*, Biblical Theology for Christian Proclamation (Nashville: B&H Publishing Group, 2015).

Senor, Thomas. "Drawing on Many Traditions: An Ecumenical Kenotic Christology," in Anna Marmadoro and Jonathan Hill, eds., *The Metaphysics of the Incarnation* (Oxford: Oxford University Press, 2011), pp. 88–113.

Sonderegger, Katherine. *Systematic Theology, Volume One: The Doctrine of God* (Minneapolis: Fortress Press, 2015).

Smith, Aaron T. "God's Self-Specification: His Being Is His Electing," in Michael T. Dempsey, ed., *Trinity and Election in Contemporary Theology* (Grand Rapids: William B. Eerdmans Publishing Co., 2011), pp. 201–225.

Sprinkle, Preston M. "Πίστις Χριστου as an Eschatological Event," in Michael F. Bird and Preston M. Sprinkle, eds., *The Faith of Jesus Christ: Exegetical, Biblical, and Theological Studies* (Peabody: Hendrickson Publishers, 2009), pp. 165–184.

Stanglin, Keith D. and Thomas H. McCall. *After Arminius: A Historical Introduction to Arminian Theology* (New York: Oxford University Press, 2020).

Stanglin, Keith D. and Thomas H. McCall. *Jacob Arminius: Theologian of Grace* (New York: Oxford University Press, 2012).

Stanley, Jason. "Names and Rigid Designation," in Bob Hale and Crispin Wright, eds., *A Companion to Philosophy of Language* (Oxford: Blackwell, 1997), pp. 555–585.

Steinmetz, David C. "The Superiority of Pre-Critical Exegesis," *Theology Today* 37:1 (1980), pp. 27–38.

Strohminger, Nina and Shaun Nichols. "The Essential Moral Self" *Cognition* 131:1 (2014), pp. 159–171.

Stump, Eleonore. *Aquinas* (New York: Routledge, 2003).

Stump, Eleonore. "Aquinas's Metaphysics of the Incarnation," in Stephen T. Davis, Daniel Kendall, S. J. and Gerald O'Collins, S. J., eds., *The Incarnation: An Interdisciplinary Symposium on the Incarnation of the Son of God* (Oxford: Oxford University Press, 2002), pp. 197–218.

Stump, Eleonore. "Omnipresence, Indwelling, and the Second-Personal," *European Journal for Philosophy of Religion* 5:4 (2013), pp. 29–53.

Stump, Eleonore. *Wandering in Darkness: Narrative and the Problem of Suffering* (Oxford: Oxford University Press, 2010).

Sumner, Darren. "Obedience and Subordination in Karl Barth's Trinitarian Theology," in Oliver D. Crisp and Fred Sanders, eds., *Advancing Trinitarian Theology: Explorations in Constructive Dogmatics* (Grand Rapids: Zondervan Academic, 2015), pp. 130–146.

Swain, Scott R. *The God of the Gospel: Robert Jenson's Trinitarian Theology* (Downers Grove: InterVarsity Academic, 2013).

Swinburne, Richard. *The Christian God* (Oxford: Oxford University Press, 1994).

Tanner, Kathryn. *Christ the Key* (Cambridge: Cambridge University Press, 2010).

Tarzi, Paul Nadim. *Galatians: A Commentary* (Crestwood, NY: St. Vladimir's Seminary Press, 1994).

Thiselton, Anthony C. "Speech-Act Theory and the Claim that God Speaks: Nicholas Wolterstorff's *Divine Discourse*," *Scottish Journal of Theology* 50:1 (1997), pp. 97–110.

Thompson, Marianne Meye. *The God of the Gospel of John* (Grand Rapids: William B. Eerdmans Publishing Co., 2001).

Thompson, Marianne Meye. *John: A Commentary* (Louisville: Westminster John Knox Press, 2015).

Thompson, Thomas R. "Trinitarianism Today: Doctrinal Renaissance, Ethical Relevance, Social Redolence," *Calvin Theological Journal* 32:1 (1997), pp. 9–42.

Tilling, Chris. "Campbell's Faith: Advancing the *Pistis Christou* Debate," in Chris Tilling, ed., *Beyond Old and New Perspectives on Paul: Reflections on the Work of Douglas Campbell* (Eugene: Cascade Books, 2014), pp. 234–250.

Tilling, Chris. *Paul's Divine Christology* (Grand Rapids: William B. Eerdmans Publishing Co., 2015).

Torrance, Thomas F. *The Christian Doctrine of God: One Being, Three Persons* (Edinburgh: T&T Clark, 1996).

Torrance, Thomas F. *Karl Barth: Biblical and Evangelical Theologian* (Edinburgh: T&T Clark, 2001).

Torrance, Thomas F. "One Aspect of the Biblical Conception of Faith," *Expository Times* 68:4 (1957), pp. 111–114.

Torrance, Thomas F. *The Trinitarian Faith: The Evangelical Theology of the Ancient Catholic Church* (Edinburgh: T&T Clark, 1988).

Treier, Daniel J. *Introducing Theological Interpretation of Scripture: Recovering a Christian Practice* (Grand Rapids: Baker Academic, 2008).

Turretin, Francis. *Institutes of Elenctic Theology: Volume Two*, trans. George Musgrave Giger, ed. James T. Dennison, Jr. (Philipsburg, NJ: Presbyterian and Reformed, 1992).

Turretin, Francis. *Institutio Theologiae Elencticae, Pars Secunda XVII.III* (Geneva, 1582).

van Driel, Edwin Chr. "Karl Barth on the Eternal Existence of Jesus Christ," *Scottish Journal of Theology* 60:1 (2007), pp. 45–61.

Vanhoozer, Kevin J. *Remythologizing Theology: Divine Action, Passion, and Authorship* (Cambridge: Cambridge University Press, 2010).

Vanhoye, Albert. *Old Testament Priests and the New Priest According to the New Testament* (Petersham, MA: St. Bede's Publications, 1986).

Vanhoye, Albert. *Structure and Message of the Epistle to the Hebrews* (Rome: Editrice Pontifico Instituto Biblico, 1989).

van Inwagen, Peter. "Critical Studies of the New Testament and the User of the New Testament," in Thomas P. Flint and Eleonore Stump, eds., *Hermes and Athena: Biblical Exegesis and Philosophical Theology* (Notre Dame: University of Notre Dame Press, 1993), pp. 159–190.

van Inwagen, Peter. *God, Knowledge, and Mystery: Essays in Philosophical Theology* (Ithaca: Cornell University Press, 1995).

van Mastricht, Petrus. *Theoretico-Practiica Theologia, editio secunda VI.VIII.XXVII* (Utrecht, 1698).

Voetius, Gisbert. *Thersites Heautontimorenos hoc est Remonstrantum Hyperaspistes* (Utrecht, 1635).

Wallis, Ian G. *The Faith of Jesus Christ in Early Christian Traditions* (Cambridge: Cambridge University Press, 1995).

Walton, John. *The Lost World of Adam and Eve: Genesis 2–3 and the Human Origins Debate* (Downers Grove: InterVarsity Academic, 2015).

Ward, Keith. *Christ and the Cosmos: A Reformulation of Trinitarian Doctrine* (Cambridge: Cambridge University Press, 2015).

Ward, Keith. "Reimagining the Trinity: On Not Three Gods," *Philosophia Christi* 18:2 (2016).

Watson, Francis. *Paul and the Hermeneutics of Faith*, second edition (New York: Bloomsbury T&T Clark, 2016).

Watson, Francis. *Text and Truth* (Grand Rapids: William B. Eerdmans Publishing Co., 1997).

Webb, Stephen H. *Jesus Christ, Eternal God: Heavenly Flesh and the Metaphysics of Matter* (Oxford: Oxford University Press, 2012).

Webster, John B. "One Who is Son: Theological Reflections on the Exordium to the Epistle to the Hebrews," in Richard Bauckham, Daniel R. Driver, Trevor A. Hart, and Nathan MacDonald, eds., *The Epistle to the Hebrews and Christian Theology* (Grand Rapids: William B. Eerdmans Publishing Co., 2009), pp. 69–94.

Webster, John B. "Principles of Systematic Theology," *International Journal of Systematic Theology* 11:1 (2009), pp. 56–71.

Wesley, John. "Address to the Clergy," in *The Works of John Wesley, Volume X: Letters, Essays, Dialogs, and Addresses* (Grand Rapids: Zondervan, n.d.), pp. 480–500.

Westerholm, Stephen. *Perspectives Old and New on Paul: The "Lutheran" Paul and His Critics* (Grand Rapids: William B. Eerdmans Publishing Co., 2004).

White, Thomas Joseph, O. P., *The Incarnate Lord: A Thomistic Study in Christology* (Washington: Catholic University of America Press, 2015).

Wiggins, David. *Sameness and Substance* (Oxford: Blackwell, 1980).

Willard, Dallas. "Jesus the Logician," *Christian Scholars Review* XXVIII:4 (1999), pp. 605–614.

Wiley, H. Orton. *The Epistle to the Hebrews* (Kansas City: Beacon Hill Press, 1959).

Williams, Sam. "Again *Pistis Christou*," *Catholic Biblical Quarterly* 49 (1987), pp. 431–447.

Williams, Scott. "In Defense of a Latin Social Trinity: A Response to William Hasker," *Faith and Philosophy* (2010), pp. 96–117.

Williams, Scott. "Indexicals and the Trinity: Two Non-Social Models," *Journal of Analytic Theology* 1 (2013), pp. 74–94.

Witherington III, Ben. *Biblical Theology: The Convergence of the Canon* (Cambridge: Cambridge University Press, 2019).

Witherington III, Ben. *Grace in Galatia: A Commentary on Paul's Letter to the Galatians* (Edinburgh: T&T Clark, 1998).

Witherington III, Ben. *Letters and Homilies for Jewish Christians: A Socio-Rhetorical Commentary on Hebrews, James and Jude* (Downers Grove: InterVarsity Academic, 2007).

Wollebius, Johannes. *Christianae theologiae compendium* (Amsterdam, 1655).

Wolterstorff, Nicholas. *Divine Discourse: Philosophical Reflections on the Claim that God Speaks* (Cambridge: Cambridge University Press, 1995).

Wolterstorff, Nicholas. "Is There Justice in the Trinity?" in Miroslav Volf and Michael Welker, eds., *God's Life in Trinity* (Minneapolis: Fortress Press, 2006), pp. 177–187.

Wolterstorff, Nicholas. "To Theologians: From One Who Cares About Theology but Is Not One of You," *Theological Education* 40:2 (2005), pp. 79–92.

Wright, N. T. "Five Gospels but No Gospel: Jesus and the Seminar," in Bruce Chilton and Craig Evans, eds., *Authenticating the Activities of Jesus: New Testament Tools and Studies* (Leiden: Brill, 1999).

Wright, N. T. "Jesus and the Identity of God," *Ex Auditu* 14 (1998), pp. 42–56.

Wright, N. T. *Jesus and the Victory of God: Christian Origins and the Question of God, Volume Two* (Minneapolis: Fortress Press, 1996).

Wright, N. T. *Paul and the Faithfulness of God* (Minneapolis: Fortress Press, 2013).

Wright, N. T. *Paul and His Recent Interpreters: Some Contemporary Debates* (Minneapolis: Fortress Press, 2015).

Yandell, Keith E. *The Epistemology of Religious Experience* (Cambridge: Cambridge University Press, 1993).

Yandell, Keith E. "Divine Necessity and Divine Goodness," in Thomas V. Morris, ed., *Divine and Human Action: Essays in the Metaphysics of Theism* (Ithaca: Cornell University Press, 1988), pp. 313–344.

Yaqub, Alladin M. *An Introduction to Logical Theory* (Buffalo: Broadview Press, 2013).

Zanchi, Hieronymous. *De Natura Dei, Seu De Divinis Attributis* (Nuestadt, 1593).

Ziegler, Philip G. *Militant Grace: The Apocalyptic Turn and the Future of Christian Theology* (Grand Rapids: Baker Academic, 2018).

Zizioulas, John D. *Being as Communion: Studies in Personhood and the Church* (Crestwood, NY: St. Vladimir's Seminary Press, 1985).

Index